LIVING

DR TOM SMITH spent six years in general practice and seven years in medical research before taking up writing full time in 1977. He writes regularly for medical journals and magazines and has a weekly column in the Scottish *Sunday Mail* and the *Bradford Telegraph and Argus*. He is the author of *Living with High Blood Pressure*, *Coping with Strokes*, *Coping with Bronchitis and Emphysema* and *Heart Attacks – Prevent and Survive* (all Sheldon Press). He still does some general practice in South West Scotland. He is married with two married children and three grandchildren.

Overcoming Common Problems Series

For a full list of titles please contact
Sheldon Press, Marylebone Road, London NW1 4DU

The Assertiveness Workbook
A plan for busy women
JOANNA CUTMANN

Beating the Comfort Trap
DR WINDY DRYDEN AND JACK
GORDON

Birth Over Thirty Five
SHEILA KITZINGER

Body Language
How to read others' thoughts by their
gestures
ALLAN PEASE

Body Language in Relationships
DAVID COHEN

Calm Down
How to cope with frustration and anger
DR PAUL HAUCK

Cancer – A Family Affair
NEVILLE SHONE

Comfort for Depression
JANET HORWOOD

Coping Successfully with Hayfever
DR ROBERT YOUNGSON

Coping Successfully with Migraine
SUE DYSON

Coping Successfully with Pain
NEVILLE SHONE

Coping Successfully with PMS
KAREN EVENNETT

Coping Successfully with Panic Attacks
SHIRLEY TRICKETT

**Coping Successfully with Prostrate
Problems**
ROSY REYNOLDS

**Coping Successfully with Your
Hyperactive Child**
DR PAUL CARSON

**Coping Successfully with Your Irritable
Bowel**
ROSEMARY NICOL

**Coping Successfully with Your Second
Child**
FIONA MARSHALL

Coping with Anxiety and Depression
SHIRLEY TRICKETT

Coping with Blushing
DR ROBERT EDELMANN

Coping with Bronchitis and Emphysema
DR TOM SMITH

Coping with Candida
SHIRLEY TRICKETT

Coping with Chronic Fatigue
TRUDIE CHALDER

Coping with Cot Death
SARAH MURPHY

Coping with Crushes
ANITA NAIK

Coping with Cystitis
CAROLINE CLAYTON

Coping with Depression and Elation
DR PATRICK McKEON

Coping with Postnatal Depression
FIONA MARSHALL

Coping with Psoriasis
PROFESSOR RONALD MARKS

Coping with Schizophrenia
DR STEVEN JONES AND DR FRANK
TALLIS

Coping with Strokes
DR TOM SMITH

Coping with Suicide
DR DONALD SCOTT

Coping with Thyroid Problems
DR JOAN GOMEZ

Coping with Thrush
CAROLINE CLAYTON

Curing Arthritis Exercise Book
MARGARET HILLS AND JANET
HORWOOD

Overcoming Common Problems Series

Curing Arthritis Diet Book
MARGARET HILLS

Curing Arthritis – The Drug-Free Way
MARGARET HILLS

Curing Arthritis
More ways to a drug-free life
MARGARET HILLS

Curing Illness – The Drug-Free Way
MARGARET HILLS

Depression
DR PAUL HAUCK

Divorce and Separation
Every woman's guide to a new life
ANGELA WILLANS

Don't Blame Me!
How to stop blaming yourself and other people
TONY GOUGH

Everything Parents Should Know About Drugs
SARAH LAWSON

Family First Aid and Emergency Handbook
DR ANDREW STANWAY

Getting Along with People
DIANNE DOUBTFIRE

Getting the Best for Your Bad Back
DR ANYTHONY CAMPBELL

Good Stress Guide, The
MARY HARTLEY

Heart Attacks – Prevent and Survive
DR TOM SMITH

Helping Children Cope with Bullying
SARAH LAWSON

Helping Children Cope with Divorce
ROSEMARY WELLS

Helping Children Cope with Grief
ROSEMARY WELLS

Hold Your Head Up High
DR PAUL HAUCK

How to Be Your Own Best Friend
DR PAUL HAUCK

How to Cope when the Going Gets Tough
DR WINDY DRYDEN AND JACK GORDON

How to Cope with Bulimia
DR JOAN GOMEZ

How to Cope with Difficult People
ALAN HOUEL WITH CHRISTIAN GODEFROY

How to Cope with Splitting Up
VERA PEIFFER

How to Cope with Stress
DR PETER TYRER

How to Cope with your Child's Allergies
DR PAUL CARSON

How to Do What You Want to Do
DR PAUL HAUCK

How to Improve Your Confidence
DR KENNETH HAMBLY

How to Interview and Be Interviewed
MICHELE BROWN AND GYLES BRANDRETH

How to Keep Your Cholesterol in Check
DR ROBERT POVEY

How to Love and Be Loved
DR PAUL HAUCK

How to Pass Your Driving Test
DONALD RIDLAND

How to Stand up for Yourself
DR PAUL HAUCK

How to Start a Conversation and Make Friends
DON GABOR

How to Stop Smoking
GEORGE TARGET

How to Stop Worrying
DR FRANK TALLIS

How to Survive Your Teenagers
SHEILA DAINOW

How to Untangle Your Emotional Knots
DR WINDY DRYDEN AND JACK GORDON

How to Write a Successful CV
JOANNA GUTMANN

Overcoming Common Problems Series

Hysterectomy
SUZIE HAYMAN

Is HRT Right for You?
DR ANNE MACGREGOR

The Incredible Sulk
DR WINDY DRYDEN

The Irritable Bowel Diet Book
ROSEMARY NICOL

The Irritable Bowel Stress Book
ROSEMARY NICOL
Jealousy
DR PAUL HAUCK

Learning to Live with Multiple Sclerosis
DR ROBERT POVEY, ROBIN DOWIE
AND GILLIAN PRETT

Living Through Personal Crisis
ANN KAISER STEARNS

Living with Asthma
DR ROBERT YOUNGSON

Living with Diabetes
DR JOAN GOMEZ

Living with Grief
DR TONY LAKE

Living with High Blood Pressure
DR TOM SMITH

Making the Most of Loving
GILL COX AND SHEILA DAINOW

Making the Most of Yourself
GILL COX AND SHEILA DAINOW

Menopause
RAEWYN MACKENZIE

Migraine Diet Book, The
SUE DYSON

Motor Neurone Disease – A Family Affair
DR DAVID OLIVER

The Nervous Person's Companion
DR KENNETH HAMBLY

Overcoming Guilt
DR WINDY DRYDEN

Overcoming Stress
DR VERNON COLEMAN

The Parkinson's Disease Handbook
DR RICHARD GODWIN-AUSTEN

Sleep Like a Dream – The Drug-Free Way
ROSEMARY NICOL

Subfertility Handbook, The
VIRGINIA IRONSIDE AND SARAH
BIGGS

Talking About Anorexia
How to cope with life without starving
MAROUSHKA MONRO

Talking About Miscarriage
SARAH MURPHY

Ten Steps to Positive Living
DR WINDY DRYDEN

Think Your Way to Happiness
DR WINDY DRYDEN AND JACK
GORDON

**Understanding Obsessions and
Compulsions**
A self-help manual
DR FRANK TALLIS

Understanding Your Personality
Myers-Briggs and more
PATRICIA HEDGES

A Weight Off Your Mind
How to stop worrying about your body size
SUE DYSON

When your Child Comes Out
ANNE LOVELL

You and Your Varicose Veins
DR PATRICIA GILBERT

Overcoming Common Problems

LIVING WITH ANGINA

Dr Tom Smith

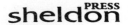
sheldon PRESS

First published in Great Britain in 1996 .
Sheldon Press, SPCK, Marylebone Road, London NW1 4DU

Illustrations by Alasdair J.D. Smith

British Library Cataloguing-in-Publication Data
A catalogue record for this book is available
from the British Library

ISBN 0–85969–749–5 ✓

Typeset by Deltatype Ltd, Ellesmere Port, Cheshire
Printed in Great Britain by Biddles Ltd, Guildford and King's Lynn

Contents

	Introduction	1
1	Patterns of angina	5
2	Angina and other chest pains	13
3	Explaining angina – a question of supply and demand	17
4	Why me? Looking for the causes of angina	29
5	Reducing the risk factors – tackling cholesterol: the evidence	40
6	Reducing the risk factors – your changing lifestyle	50
7	Taking up – and keeping up – exercise	58
8	Smoking	70
9	Alcohol	81
10	High blood pressure	86
11	Managing angina – entering the heart unit	89
12	Treating angina – medicines and surgery	94
13	Women – and children	106
	Appendix 1: Useful organizations	111
	Appendix 2: Glossary	112
	Index	115

For Laura

Introduction

Pain in the chest is terrifying. The first time it hits, out of the blue, it feels like a death sentence. We assume that it must be the start of a heart attack, and we have all heard – unless we have just arrived from another planet – that heart attacks kill.

Naturally, when the pain goes away – often as suddenly as it has arrived – there is a huge sense of relief. We think that maybe it wasn't heart pain after all. It could have been indigestion, or cramp in a chest muscle, or anything other than we feared at the time. Gradually, the anxiety ebbs away, and we think of something else. We probably don't even bother to go to the doctor.

The second time it happens, we expect it to go away – and it does, as soon as we stop doing whatever provoked it. There is less anxiety, and we carry on as we were.

It is usually only after the third or fourth bout of pain in the chest that we decide to go to the doctor. Even then, we probably don't bring up in conversation with the doctor the possibility that heart trouble may be at the root of the pain. But deep down the fear is there – and when it is confirmed, life is never the same again. Once the pain has been labelled 'angina', we feel that we are living on a knife edge – and that some day the dreaded 'heart attack' will arrive.

This book is for people who are living on that knife edge – angina sufferers and their families. It is entitled *Living with Angina* with good reason, because its message is that angina is *not* a death sentence. We can survive it, and we can do a lot to help ourselves to do so.

People with angina are by no means alone. Proof of that, if it were needed, comes from the British Regional Heart Study, which started in 1978. Since then, family doctors in 24 towns in England, Scotland and Wales have been following 7,735 men who were aged 40–59 in 1978. The men were chosen at random from the practice registers, regardless of their health.

A staggering 8 per cent of the men approached in the study admitted to chest pains on exercise that were later confirmed as

1

angina as a result of heart disease. Yet even when that pain had been severe, 40 per cent of them could not recall that their doctors had made a 'heart' diagnosis.

Even more disturbing, when the 7,735 men underwent full questioning and electrocardiography, a quarter of them showed some evidence that they had heart disease that would lead eventually to angina – and were consequently at higher than normal risk of a heart attack.

How high this risk was is shown by the current figures for heart attacks among the 7,735 men. In the group with chest pains at the start of the study, there have been more than twice as many heart attacks as in those who had no chest pains. In the group with angina and a probable previous heart attack (they admitted to at least one bout of very severe chest pain lasting longer than usual, even at rest), there have since been six times more heart attacks than in the others.

The heart attacks they have had are the 'endpoints' (the word used by the researchers) of angina (its full medical term is *angina pectoris*). This book explains what angina is, and why so many of us have it. By describing the physical background to the disease, it should help to take the mystique and fear out of it, allowing sufferers to minimize and manage their own attacks without panic, and to do all they can to avoid their own 'endpoint'.

Living with Angina explains how doctors approach the investigation and treatment of angina, with drugs and surgery – both of which are very much more successful than they were, and still continue to improve. Throughout, we concentrate on the three principal contributors to angina – cigarette smoking, high blood pressure and high blood cholesterol levels. Also, the book tackles the contributions to angina made by heredity, stress, obesity, lack of exercise and alcohol.

However, this book does *not* recommend a specific diet. In books, magazines and television programmes we have been swamped with advice (and often it is more like propaganda) on what we should eat to keep the heart and circulation healthy. The food companies have been hammering away at the 'butter or margarine', 'red meat versus fish', and 'high fibre versus sugar' debates for years, with little effect on the health of the nation.

These debates have reached their heights in the United States, where, despite the very strong messages put out by the 'good health' lobby, the population has been getting fatter by the year. If the present trend continues, 100 per cent of Americans will be obese by the year 2230!

Of course, that will not happen, for there will always be some people who will heed the 'good health' messages. One aim of this book is to persuade *you* to do so.

The 'health message' pervades the whole of *Living with Angina*, but the last chapters, on the modern treatment of angina pectoris, are very important for all angina sufferers. In recent years, the medical treatment of angina has become very complex, and many angina sufferers are understandably confused by the different drugs they are asked to take and why they have to take them. Thus the final chapters describe these drugs and give the reasons for their prescription.

Yet drugs alone are only a small part of the management of angina. The main effort must come from you, the patient. Surgeons can give you what is virtually a new circulation in the heart, and doctors can give you medicines that will ease the pain of angina, take the strain from the heart, improve its circulation and its rhythm, and make you feel better. But if you don't also make the effort to live healthily, then all these doctors' efforts may well be in vain.

If the thought of living healthily makes you groan, don't stop reading! Changing your lifestyle is no great bind – in fact, it can even be fun. Eating differently means enjoying new tastes. Stopping smoking adds to that by heightening your sense of taste. Finding ways to exercise can be great fun. Losing a stone or two makes you feel years younger. Feeling as fit as you can be, perhaps for the first time in years, can help you find the sort of joy in living you had as a child. So please read on!

1

Patterns of angina

Jim

Jim is 41 years old, and a friend of mine. He signed on as a patient in our practice three years ago, when he moved into the district. A freelance graphic designer, Jim had welcomed the move from the city to our rural idyll in the west of Scotland, seeing it as a haven of peace in which he could get down to his work with little interruption.

When Jim arrived in our district, he decided to take advantage of the country walks to lose the excess weight he'd put on and get in trim – for he was aware that he had been neglecting his fitness. Things went well for a week or two, but then he became a little more adventurous. Few roads in the west of Scotland are flat for any distance, so soon he started to tackle the gentle hills.

It was then that Jim came to the surgery, complaining of 'indigestion'. It seemed that during a walk he would often get a tight feeling in the centre of his chest that would only go away if he rested for a while. Sometimes it was an actual pain, dull and aching, deep within his chest, that travelled as far as his upper left arm or into the left side of his lower jaw. It mostly started when walking up an incline, but it could also affect him on the flat. The pain always went away within a few seconds if he stopped walking, and even faster if he sat down.

The pain didn't worry Jim: he thought it was probably some form of muscle cramp, and asked if we could prescribe some tablets for it.

Tablets were not the first thing in our minds! This story of a pain or tightness in the chest on exertion that goes away at rest must be considered as angina due to coronary heart disease until proved otherwise. And in a man as young as 41, any possibility of angina must be taken seriously.

Jim had never been ill in his life, he said, except for a bout of 'pleurisy' at age 36 when he was abroad. On further questioning, though, his 'pleurisy' had been mainly an illness of severe chest pain and breathlessness. His doctor of that time had told him to stay in bed, at home, for two weeks, given him antibiotics, and then let him go back to work. Jim had felt awful for a month or two afterwards, but gradually returned to normal. He had the feeling, though, that he had never been 'quite the same man' since this illness.

My colleagues and I were not surprised, for his electrocardiogram (ECG) showed that he had had a heart attack in the past – and that the bout of 'pleurisy' had probably been that attack.

We put Jim on a 'treadmill' and tested his ECG again. As we asked him to walk faster, and increased the upward slope of the platform on which he was walking, we saw the changes we expected. There was evidence that his heart was not getting enough oxygen for the work it was being expected to do: shortly after the change in the ECG appeared, so did the pain.

We stopped the test, let him rest, then explained that he had angina, which needed treatment. Because he was only 41, and there was evidence of a previous heart attack, we referred Jim to our local specialist cardiology unit (unit dealing with heart problems). There, an angiogram, which is a picture showing the inside of the arteries, showed that he had narrowed sites in all three main coronary arteries, and he was placed on the waiting list for bypass surgery.

In the meantime, we took Jim's lifestyle in hand! We told him that he had to stop smoking straight away (he smoked ten cigarettes a day). He also had to eat less, and change to a diet low in animal fats (his blood cholesterol level – level of fat in the blood – was slightly above normal). We suggested he switch to a 'Mediterranean'-type diet, which means plenty of fruit and vegetables, seafood and pasta. He could have the odd glass of red wine in the evening with his meal, but he needed to avoid excess alcohol, red meats and full-cream dairy products. We told him he should exercise as much as he could, up to the point of experiencing pain. Once he was in pain, he was always to stop immediately and rest until the pain subsided completely.

Jim was given glyceryl trinitrate tablets to place under his tongue when the pain started, and even to use before he knew he was going for an energetic walk. He was also asked to take half an adult aspirin a day, permanently. His blood pressure was on the high side, so he was given pills called 'beta-blockers' to reduce it, and was asked to return to have it measured once a week for the next month or so.

After just one week, the change in Jim was astonishing. He was able to walk three times as far as he had previously, before the pain started, and the treadmill showed that he could tolerate much more exercise still. He lost a little weight, and his blood pressure had fallen into the normal range. In fact, Jim felt so much better that he asked if his impending operation was really necessary. We thought that it was, because he was still relatively young, and we were still worried about those nasty narrowings in his coronary arteries.

Two months after he saw us for the first time, Jim had his bypass operation. His arteries were ragged from a condition called atheroma (see Chapter 3), and he needed three different bypasses, using grafts from branches of an artery inside the chest wall, to get round the worst of the narrowed areas.

He recovered remarkably quickly from the surgery, and in the three years since his operation, he has never smoked a cigarette, he has got his weight down to normal, and has even started jogging. In fact, Jim aims to complete the Great Scottish Run – the annual half-marathon around the streets of Glasgow, which attracts some 7,000 runners – next year. I'm sure he will. He no longer has chest pains, even when he jogs. Since he lost the weight, his blood pressure has remained normal, and is now even on the low side, so that he has stopped his drugs, except for the aspirin, which he accepts he will take for the rest of his life.

Jim is the model patient. Once his illness was spelled out for him, he determined to look after himself. He was not only doing it for himself, but for his wife and two children. As a self-employed man still in his forties, he knows only too well that they might be left alone, with very little behind them financially, if he were not to heed the warnings of his heart.

John Hunter

Jim should prove more fortunate than my second example of angina, John Hunter. He was the best-known surgeon of the eighteenth century. A Scot who took the high road to London, he developed angina in his fifties. He told his colleagues that his life was 'in the hands of any rascal who chose to annoy or tease him'.

During a meeting of the Board of Governors of St George's Hospital in London in 1783, John Hunter became involved in an angry dispute with the other members of the Board. He suddenly stopped speaking, struggled to control his temper, then hurried into another room. There, according to his biographer, G. Qvist (in the book *John Hunter 1728–1783*, 1981, Heinemann), he died within a few minutes.

John Hunter did not, of course, have the advantages of today's knowledge of angina. Emotions such as anger or fear can increase the heart rate and blood pressure well beyond that to which the angina-affected heart can adjust, and the result is sudden heart failure. John Hunter's death is still a lesson to us today: that attention to the psychological and emotional state is important for anyone with angina.

James Fixx

James Fixx is my next example. He was famous in the 1970s for his book *The Art of Running* (1979, Chatto & Windus), in which he recommended exercise, and particularly running long distances, for people with angina. His book was a best-seller, and was very influential in establishing today's fashion for marathons, half-marathons and 'fun-runs', in which thousands of people take part.

For that we have to thank Mr Fixx, but sadly he became more famous still when he died during one of his runs – from a heart attack. Some people have used his premature death as an excuse for not doing exercise. 'Exercise killed Jim Fixx,' they reason, 'so it may kill me!' That is not strictly true. Exercise may have allowed James to live much longer than he otherwise would have done – but he relied too much upon it, and too little on other ways to improve his health.

The facts about James Fixx are as follows. In his mid-thirties he had a heart problem diagnosed. He weighed 16 stones (100 kilograms), and got breathless when trying to run 50 metres. He took up running, and ten years later, in 1978, he had lost 4 stones (25 kilograms), had run a distance equivalent to going around the Equator, had completed many marathons, and was running 10 miles (16 kilometres) every day.

He died in 1989, in his late fifties. James's problem was that he believed that he could 'run through' his angina, and became so engrossed in his running schedule that he did not seek help for his increasing angina. He had, in fact, severe coronary artery disease (atheroma – see Chapter 3), which was probably a left-over from his days of being overweight. His father had died of coronary artery disease in his thirties, which suggests that there might have been an inherited tendency to very high levels of fat (cholesterol) in the blood.

James Fixx made the mistake of thinking that exercise is everything – that it could reverse all the problems that his previous lifestyle (and perhaps his genes) had laid down in his coronary arteries. Unfortunately it can't. If he had slowed down a little, and asked for medical advice, he might still be alive today. Even in the 1980s, there were effective ways to reduce cholesterol levels and to improve the coronary circulation. James might well have been a good candidate for coronary bypass surgery. With better circulation through his coronary arteries, he might still be running today.

Jane

Three ladies make up my last three examples of angina. The first, Jane, is aged 60. She has been well all her life, and sailed through the menopause with no difficulty. In fact, she prided herself on having done so without the need for hormone replacement therapy. However, now that her family were grown up and away, and she and her now-retired husband had bought a smaller house near the sea, her life had become much less active. She took the odd walk, but the garden took only a few minutes a day, and she was becoming a 'couch potato'. A non-smoker and non-drinker, she ate well, and was steadily putting on weight.

Jane's extra weight was the main reason for her visit to the doctor. She was getting breathless and a little 'tight-chested' when walking up the steps to her front door, or walking over the dunes to and from the beach. She was less able than before to keep up with her husband, and this irked her. So Jane asked her doctor for a diet sheet so that she could lose weight.

The 'tight-chested' feeling worried her doctor, who ordered an ECG and various blood tests. Jane's blood pressure was normal, but her blood cholesterol level was over 9 mmol/1 – well above the average – and her ECG showed changes suspicious of ischaemia, the medical term for a lack of blood supply. A treadmill test confirmed that the 'tightness' in the chest was linked to further ECG changes that showed that one of the coronary arteries was not delivering enough oxygen to the left side of the heart.

Jane was staggered to find that this 'tightness' was, in fact, angina. The subsequent angiogram showed that she had one narrowed area in the main left coronary artery, and that the area beyond it was now being served by new 'collateral' arteries that had grown in from another coronary artery. In fact, her heart was trying to deal with the problem in its own way – by producing a 'natural bypass'.

The surgeon and cardiologist agreed that with medical treatment to keep the coronaries as open as possible, and a programme of judicious exercise and weight reduction, Jane might well get away without surgery.

She is now eating and exercising better, has lost over 2 stones in weight, has lost her attacks of tightness, and is feeling much better. Her cholesterol level is down to 7 mmol/1 – still relatively high, but not in the danger area for a woman of her age. Jane has to visit her doctor every month or so, but there is every chance she will be able to avoid surgery.

Diane

Diane was just 41 when her coronary disease was discovered – and she had no pain at all. She has had diabetes since she was a child, for which she has had to self-inject insulin three times a day. There was a time in her teenage years when she 'went a little wild' and let her control slip – a natural reaction at that age to the restrictions of diabetes. However, for the last 20 years she had kept her diabetes under reasonable control.

In the last year or so, though, Diane has not been feeling well, especially when trying to look after her two children. Like many career women today, she started her family late, so that her two boys are aged six and four – *and* quite a handful.

As with many women with diabetes who become pregnant in their thirties, Diane had a difficult time. Her diabetes was hard to control, particularly near the end of each pregnancy, and the effort of bringing up the two children exhausted her. Her husband did the best he could, but he eventually forced her to see her doctor when it was obvious that she could not cope.

The story of exhaustion alerted Diane's doctors. Most women are protected from the effects of heart disease during their reproductive years by their hormones. The monthly cycle of hormonal changes in some way (we do not yet know how) postpones the onset of heart disease in women, and it is only after the menopause that they seem to develop this disease. However, the exception is in women with diabetes. Diabetes appears to neutralize the protective effect of the female hormones, so that women with diabetes are at just as much risk of angina as men of the same age.

There is, however, one striking difference. Angina in women with diabetes is often painless. With diabetes comes a condition called diabetic cardiac neuropathy, or DCN. The name simply means that, in diabetes, the nerves that convey pain to the brain from the heart are altered. The nerves no longer relay the sensation of pain, so that angina is 'silent'. The lack of oxygen is not perceived in pain, but it may appear instead as a general malaise or simply exhaustion.

This was the case for Diane. An angiogram showed that she, like the first patient, Jim, had several narrowed segments in all three main coronary arteries. She was given a priority waiting-list place for bypass surgery, and was called in for surgery a month later. However, she was also referred to her specialist in diabetes for intensive control of her glucose and insulin levels, so that she would be as fit as possible for the operation.

The surgery was a great success. When coronary artery bypass surgery was first started in the early 1970s, there were doubts about whether people with diabetes would do as well as non-diabetics. These doubts have now been dispelled, following the analysis of the results of large series of patients (in which around one in ten have had diabetes). Through surgery, angina can be considerably improved, whether it is 'silent' or painful, in people with diabetes.

The surgery was not the only change in Diane's life. She now has a much better lifestyle: she eats smaller meals at shorter intervals than before, and combines them with a different schedule of insulin injections, with the aim of keeping both her insulin and glucose levels as normal as possible throughout the day and night. She also has a regular check on her blood pressure, which is maintained at the lower limit of normal. (Because people with diabetes are particularly liable to angina, there is a section devoted to this later in the book.)

11

Rosemary

Rosemary, at 45, is the 'odd one out' of my six angina patients. She had symptoms indistinguishable from the others, with pain in the centre of her chest when she exerted herself, that subsided quickly when she stopped. However, the angiogram showed she had absolutely smooth coronary arteries, with no sign of a blockage in them.

It transpired that Rosemary's problem was not in the arteries themselves, but in the blood they carried to the heart. This was because, to our surprise (because she did not look particularly pale), she had very severe anaemia. Her haemoglobin level – a measure of how many oxygen-carrying red blood cells were in her bloodstream – was, at 5G/litre, only a third of normal. The red blood cells were also much larger than normal, a finding that pointed to a disorder called pernicious anaemia. This is a condition in which the body is deficient in vitamin B12. Further blood tests confirmed our suspicions, and she was put on injections of the vitamin she lacked.

As is usually the case in pernicious anaemia, Rosemary felt much better after the first injection, but it took some weeks before her blood count was back to normal. By that time, her angina had disappeared. Rosemary will need vitamin B12 injections for the rest of her life, but we consider her case to be a 'cure', at least of her angina.

Rosemary did have one thing in common with the other angina sufferers: she was unable to supply enough oxygen to satisfy her heart's demand for it. In her case, this was because, with her lack of red blood cells, the blood flowing through her normal arteries was simply unable to carry enough oxygen for her needs. In the other cases, there were plenty of red cells to flow through their circulation, but their arteries were narrowed by a disease process that was common to them all – atheroma. This failure to supply enough oxygen for the heart's demands is fundamental to an understanding of angina, and is explained more fully in Chapter 3.

2

Angina and other chest pains

Angina is simply the medical word for pain. *Angina pectoris* means pain in the chest, and the two words have slipped into common usage as meaning heart pain.

However, many pains in the chest are unconnected with the heart. They may arise from cramp or bruising in the muscles of the chest wall, or from inflammation of the surface of the lung, or from spasm or acid in the oesophagus (the gullet). A very common chest pain arises from the ribs, which can be inflamed at the junction between their bony back two-thirds and their cartilaginous front third. Coughing can bruise the muscles between the ribs, giving pain on deep breathing. Pain in the chest can even be 'referred' from the stomach, as in indigestion – although it should never be diagnosed as such until heart pain has been ruled out.

How can I tell if I've got angina?

So when you complain about chest pain to your doctor, be prepared to answer some very pertinent questions, such as the following ones: Exactly where is the pain? What does it feel like? What brings it on? How long does it last? Does anything you do relieve it? Can you do anything to prevent it? Being able to supply answers to these questions can put your doctor well on the way to a diagnosis before the examination even starts.

Pains emanating from the heart have their own special characteristics, and if you describe your pain in one of the following ways, it will raise your doctor's suspicions that you may have angina:

- Tightness around the chest
- Pressure inside my chest
- A weight on my chest
- Constriction around my chest
- An ache, like toothache

- A dull pain
- A squeezing feeling
- Crushing
- A band around my chest
- A tightness that makes me breathless
- 'It's just sore'

Other descriptions of the pain, like these below, will tend to make your doctor suspect another cause:

- A sharp pain
- Like a knife
- It comes in stabs
- Pins and needles
- It shoots across my chest
- It's worse when you press on the spot
- It's worse when I change position
- I can walk around all day with it
- It lasts all day, even when I'm resting

The precise site of the pain is very relevant. The heart is in the centre-left of the chest, but heart pain is not confined to this area. It mainly occurs behind the breastbone (in the centre of the chest) and around and above the left nipple, but it can spread up to the left shoulder, into the left half of the jaw, down into the left arm, into the back, and even into the upper abdomen. It is less likely to cross over into the right-hand side of the chest, and it is very rare for it to be entirely right-sided. (However, I did once meet a patient with entirely right-sided angina pectoris. He was a 'mirror-image' twin, whose organs were 'transposed' (on the opposite side of the body to normal), so that his heart was right-sided, and his liver and appendix were on his left side. His twin had his organs on the normal side of the body – they had developed from a single egg that had split early on in the pregnancy.)

What brings on angina?

What brings on the pain? Most angina starts with exercise. Physical effort brings it on, and rest relieves it. Your doctor will wish to know how much exercise is needed to produce the pain, and how long it lasts after you start to rest. *see patients*

Angina is graded according to how much exercise you can take before the pain starts, so try to estimate how many stairs you can climb, how far you can walk on the flat, or up a slope, or whether you can run for a bus, or dig the garden, or strain at the toilet, or make love. Don't hesitate to list *all* the times you have noticed the pain: your doctor will not be embarrassed.

For a few people, angina comes on while they are resting, or even wakes them out of a sleep. This is a serious sign, and needs urgent assessment in a specialist hospital department. Prompt investigation and treatment can prevent an imminent heart attack. The same goes for angina that doesn't go away immediately you rest, or keeps returning several times a day. If your pain is coming more often than it was, see your doctor immediately.

The next question is: What do you do when the pain starts? Do you try to walk through it, or stop until it goes away? The correct answer is ALWAYS to stop, and let it subside completely. The pain is a sign that the heart is trying to cope with an imbalance between the supply of oxygen to the heart muscle and the oxygen needed for it to fulfil the demands on it for energy. That is explained in detail in Chapter 3. Suffice it to say here that this imbalance must be corrected quickly if damage to the heart muscle is to be avoided – and the fastest way to do that is to rest. Resting quickly eases the demands made on the heart.

When the demand of the heart for oxygen exceeds the supply, the condition is called ischaemia – the medical term for lack of blood to an organ. Because of this, angina is sometimes given the label of 'ischaemic heart disease'.

If your answers to the previous questions suggest to your doctor that you have angina, the next step is investigation. Gone are the days when you would be handed a few pills to put under your tongue and told to live with the pain. If angina is suspected, the cause must be determined and, if possible, treated. Thus there will be routine blood tests to rule out problems such as anaemia, there will be different electrocardiographic tests, including 24-hour monitoring and tread-mill tests, to pinpoint defects in the coronary artery system and the extent of any ischaemia, there may be radio-isotope or echocardio-graphic tests to show how the heart muscle is beating, and finally an angiogram to see if bypass surgery is feasible.

All these tests will be described in Chapter 11. But before we move on to that, we need an explanation of how the heart works and what happens in angina.

3

Explaining angina – a question of supply and demand

How the heart works

Your heart is simply a pump, and its workings are shown in Figures 1 and 2. The left side of the heart pumps blood through your body; the right side pumps blood through your lungs. The principle is very easy to understand. Oxygen is picked up by the blood going through the lungs, and distributed to the tissues, where it is used to 'burn up' glucose to give us energy. The waste product of that energy, carbon dioxide, is picked up by the veins, carried to the right side of the heart, where it is pumped to the lungs and exchanged for more oxygen.

These are the bald facts, but they can give us no possible idea of how the heart carries out its job. No mechanical pump could perform as efficiently as the heart. No engineer can yet make a pump that acts around 70 times a minute for more than 70 years, meanwhile maintaining and repairing itself, supplying its own fuel – and not once, in all that time, breaking down or stopping for a rest!

In fact, there is no other muscle in the body like the heart. See how long you can continue to use your hand muscles without stopping. Grip a soft rubber ball in your stronger hand and squeeze it and relax just a little faster than once a second. Keep going for as long as you can. If you can manage five minutes before you tire then this is a good score. A trained athlete might last 30 minutes or more. Think of doing it day and night, without rest or sleep, for 70 years!

Yet that is what the heart does, all through our lives. Most of us never give it a second thought, but people who become aware of their heart beating can become neurotic about it, and their lives can be ruined. The first man-made heart valves used to 'ping' with every beat, and their owners could hear it plainly, especially when everything was quiet at night. It was, to say the least, disturbing.

Never giving the heart a thought, however, has its downside. Taking it completely for granted can mean that we let it become unhealthy. The more we understand about our heart, the better we can

17

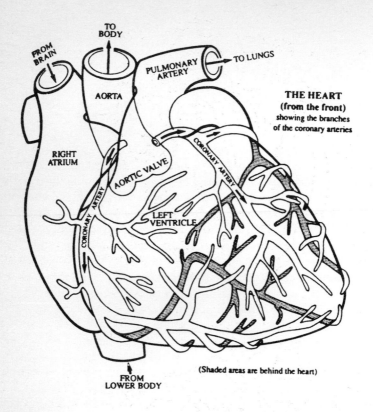

FROM BRAIN

TO BODY

PULMONARY ARTERY — TO LUNGS

AORTA

THE HEART
(from the front)
showing the branches
of the coronary arteries

RIGHT ATRIUM

CORONARY ARTERY

AORTIC VALVE

CORONARY ARTERY

LEFT VENTRICLE

CORONARY ARTERY

FROM LOWER BODY

(Shaded areas are behind the heart)

Figure 1

take care of it, and the less frightened we should be if things start to go wrong.

The first thing to understand is that the heart is a muscle, the myocardium (*myo* = muscle, *cardia* = heart). It differs from all other muscles in the body in its astonishing ability to recover extremely fast from its previous contraction or 'beat'. It completes its cycle of shortening and lengthening within a fifth of a second, then has three- or four-fifths of a second to recover, to enable it to contract again.

In that vital resting time, the heart muscle reorganizes itself so that it can shorten again without tiring. In 'beating', it uses oxygen taken

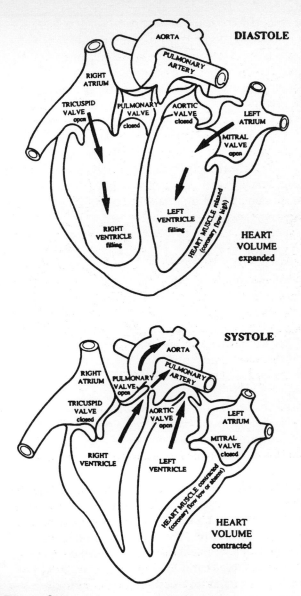

Figure 2

from the blood to convert the glucose within its stores into the energy needed for the contraction. In the rest between beats, each muscle fibre must take up more oxygen and glucose from the blood to replace the amounts lost in the previous contraction, and prepare them for the next contraction.

This constant flow of oxygen and glucose from bloodstream to myocardium is essential to life. Without them, the heart complains – and it usually does that via pain. And if the supply of oxygen and glucose to that particular part of the myocardium is not quickly restored, then that part of the muscle will die. The pain is called angina, but the death of the muscle is called 'infarction' – or, in plain language, a heart attack. Keep the supply of oxygen and glucose enough to fulfil the demands of the heart, and it will keep going for the intended 70-plus years.

What causes angina?

Angina starts when the supply of oxygen and glucose does not keep up with demand. If something impedes the easy access of oxygen and glucose to the myocardium, and the heart needs to continue beating, then it will try to find its energy source from other substances, like fats, and it will try to 'burn' them up without using oxygen. Most people when they were children have felt the results of this 'anaerobic' energy process in the 'stitch' felt in the side during running.

The pain of a stitch is caused by the accumulation of lactic acid in muscles in the side and back that have been over-used. (Fats do not 'burn' all the way down to carbon dioxide, but only get as far as lactic acid, a more complex substance, that is more difficult to remove from the tissues.)

The pain in angina has the same root. Lactic acid also builds up in a heart trying to beat without a good enough oxygen supply: the pain of angina can be similar to that of a stitch. The difference between the two is that we can tolerate a stitch, because back muscles are not so important, and eventually recover with rest. The heart muscle needs a much faster resupply of oxygen if it is to survive.

This supply of oxygen comes from the coronary arteries – so called because they form a 'crown' around the top of the heart, passing their branches over the heart surface to 'feed' the muscles that form the walls of its four chambers. In the normal heart, the three main coronary arteries and their branches are wide, strong, elastic tubes, which can expand enormously to cope with any extra flow of blood needed when the demand rises.

Naturally, this demand for a flow of blood varies hugely. When we are asleep or at complete rest, the heart rate falls to 60 per minute or below, and the blood pressure falls accordingly. At such times, the heart's demand for oxygen and glucose is low. At the opposite end of the demand spectrum are times of extreme exercise. Sprinting, whether it is to catch a train or bus, or to win the Olympic gold medal, can put up the heart's need for oxygen by 20 times or more. And if the heart is beating at or above a rate of 180 per minute, the time for recovery between beats shortens to a tenth of a second. The myocardium must be very efficient, and awash with oxygen and glucose, in order to cope with that.

Atherosclerosis (atheroma)

Unhappily, few hearts in people living in developed countries have coronary blood vessels that fulfil that ideal, and why this should be is encapsulated in one word – 'atherosclerosis'. The word 'atherosclerosis' comes from the Greek word for porridge, *atheros*. It was first used to describe patches seen in the inside surfaces of the large arteries, particularly the aorta (the main artery from the left side of the heart to the body), that look grainy, soft and crumbly – very much like porridge.

Atherosclerosis, or the short version of the word, 'atheroma', was then extended to describe the process seen inside the coronary arteries in people who have angina or who have had heart attacks. In its later stages, atheroma causes the coronary arteries to narrow, so that less blood can flow through them. It also makes them less elastic, so that they cannot expand to cope with an increased demand for blood.

If you have atheroma of the coronary arteries, the supply side of the supply-demand equation may be compromised, and the conditions for angina are established. Whether you have angina or not depends on the extent of the atheroma, and on whether there is one particular site in a coronary artery that is especially badly affected, so that the blood supply beyond it is greatly diminished.

Hardly anyone in a developed society escapes atheroma completely. American doctors examining the bodies of young soldiers killed in the Korean war were amazed by the extent of atheroma in their arteries. The first signs of this are of 'fatty streaks' in the arteries' inner surfaces, the surfaces that come into contact with the blood. Almost all of the young American soldiers possessed such streaks.

As we age, the fatty streaks become 'plaques' – plate-like thickened areas that roughen the inside surfaces of the arteries. Plaques start forming in childhood from the streaks, and grow very slowly over many years into thickened masses that protrude into the bloodstream. Their numbers and size depend almost entirely on one thing – the levels of cholesterol in the blood.

The world over, the higher the blood cholesterol level, the more extensive the atheroma. In communities existing almost entirely on fish and vegetables, such as in rural Japan, blood cholesterol levels are low, there is very little atheroma, and angina is virtually unknown. Yet Japanese people who have emigrated to the United States, and who have taken on American lifestyles, have higher cholesterol levels, and are just as prone to angina as their American neighbours.

Why should plaques be so important? We can now study the flow of blood through the coronary arteries in living people, using coronary angiography, a technique that will be explained in more detail later in the book. A 'dye' that is opaque to X-rays highlights narrowings ('stenoses') in the coronary arteries that correlate with plaque sites. Beyond the stenoses, the blood flow can be considerably reduced.

The reduction may not be much when the owner of the arteries is at rest, but the big difference comes with exercise. An artery affected by an atheromatous stenosis cannot expand to accommodate the big increase in blood flow needed when the heart is beating faster and with greater force – as in exercise or emotional stress. It may not be able to supply enough oxygen and glucose to the heart muscle that it serves, and the process leading to angina begins. The muscle must switch to anaerobic activity, lactic acid builds up, and the pain starts.

The only way to return things to normal is to reduce the heart's demand for oxygen, and the fastest way to do that is to rest.

So far, the story is clear. If we keep our cholesterol levels low, we can avoid angina. But what can we do if our coronary arteries are already affected by atheroma to the extent that we have angina? Can we reverse the process, and restore our coronary circulation to normal?

Can atherosclerosis be reversed?

The answer is that it can be, and it will take the rest of this book to explain how – with a combination of sensible eating, exercise, a different lifestyle, drugs and perhaps surgery. Yet it is important, in understanding how this can be done, to look at all the other contributors to angina, for cholesterol is not the only danger to angina sufferers.

Atheroma is the necessary background to angina, but it is hardly ever the sole cause of the symptoms. In most angina sufferers it is the combination of underlying atheroma with many other changes in the blood that causes the illness. For example, the blood may be more viscous ('sticky') than normal, slowing the flow through the stenoses. It can be more likely than normal to clot ('thrombose'). It can carry too little oxygen, perhaps because the oxygen-carrying red cells are full of carbon monoxide instead, or because of lung disease, or anaemia. All these can reduce the 'supply' side of the equation.

Or there may be high blood pressure, which, by increasing the force of the heart beat even at rest, increases the heart's demand for oxygen and glucose – causing further imbalance to the supply–demand equation.

How all these changes can combine together to create angina, and how they can all be reversed, is explained later, but in order to understand them, it is first necessary to outline the components of healthy blood.

Healthy blood

The heart should beat efficiently, be in peak condition, and have smooth, wide blood vessels that supply it with enough oxygen and glucose to deal with any demand put upon it, without clotting or

23

sticking. For this to happen, the blood itself must be in peak condition.

Blood is certainly thicker than water, and it contains within it a 'soup' of substances and cells that makes it much less than free-flowing.

First, there is the serum, the watery fluid in which all the constituents of the blood float. It carries minerals, salts and glucose, all the soluble substances needed for the continuing health of the tissues and organs, and the waste products that need disposing of through the kidneys.

Then there is the plasma, which is the name given to the serum plus a mixture of proteins and fats, mainly derived from food. Cholesterol and related fatty-protein compounds, the lipoproteins, are part of the plasma. Very fatty plasma, high in cholesterol, is more viscous than normal, it is sticky to the touch, like the stickiness left after a fry-up in a pan.

Whole blood is plasma plus the cells – the solid constituents. They include the white cells (leukocytes), which act to resist infection and inflammation; platelets, fragments of cells that initiate clotting in arteries; and the red blood cells (erythrocytes) that transport oxygen around the body.

A fluid engineer would be horrified to be asked to design a pump for a closed system of wide and narrow tubes filled with such a mixture of solid, fatty and watery substances. The difficulties in calculating the various pressures and flow rates are huge. For example, in each blood constituent – serum, plasma and cells – there are substances that can make it much more viscous. As a fluid becomes stickier, the pressure needed to push it through a small bore tube becomes very much higher, and that means a much greater effort from the heart. The demand of the myocardium for oxygen rises steeply.

Take glucose in the serum as an example. Every cell in the body needs a continuing supply of glucose to stay alive. The burning of glucose with oxygen is our main supply of energy, so the level of glucose in the blood must remain within very strict limits. If it falls too low, we become faint and weak as our muscles and brain start to fail.

However, if the blood glucose level rises too high, as it does in poorly controlled diabetes, the blood becomes measurably stickier, and thickens. This is a problem for people with diabetes, who are at higher than normal risk of angina if they do not control their glucose levels very closely for this and other reasons.

A raised glucose level, however, is a very minor change compared to a rise in blood fat levels, or if the platelets become 'stickier'. Even a small rise in fats – mainly measured as cholesterol – can make the blood much more viscous, and when this is combined with clumps (or 'aggregates') of platelets floating in the bloodstream in the smallest arteries, it can greatly reduce the smooth and easy flow of blood through them. These are changes that can happen to all of us, not just to diabetics, and which we can do much to reverse. If we let them continue, on the other hand, we are inviting the conditions for angina to develop.

The element that has the most effect on blood viscosity, or stickiness, however, is the red blood cell. Red cells, which carry the oxygen from the lungs through the heart and into the rest of the body, must be flexible, like very soft rubber, to pass through the smallest blood vessels. They are disc-like, with a diameter across the disc of around 7 microns (7 thousandths of a millimetre). The smallest capillaries (the blood vessels from which the oxygen is given up to the tissues) are only 5 to 10 microns across, so the red cells have to fold and bend to pass through them.

If the red cells become stiffer – less flexible – or pile up, almost like tubes of wine gums, into 'rouleaux', the circulation inside the capillaries becomes much less free, and the pressure needed to force the blood through the circulation has to rise. This, of course, is an extra strain on the heart.

Stiffened red cells and rouleaux can even lead to blockage of the capillaries, with thrombosis, so that the capillary circulation can even stop completely in places. This process is made worse in some people, in whom a substance promoting blood clotting, fibrinogen, is present in higher than normal amounts in the blood.

What if the red cells are not only stiffer than normal, but they also don't carry enough oxygen from the lungs? They are designed to take up oxygen in large amounts, then give it up freely when they reach the tissues. However, the red cell 'oxygen uptake' mechanism works even better for the lethal gas called carbon monoxide. Breathing in a mixture of carbon monoxide and oxygen, the red cells preferentially take up carbon monoxide, rather than oxygen – and it remains solidly bound to them, so that they can no longer take up oxygen from the lungs.

The old 'town gas' ovens used carbon monoxide, and car exhausts still contain it – and they have been a favoured method of suicide for many years. However, you don't need to breathe in a suicidal dose of carbon monoxide to do yourself harm: if you expose yourself to a small amount, day in and day out, you are giving your heart less oxygen – and reducing the supply side of the equation even further.

Changes in the blood vessel walls

So far I have listed elements within the circulating blood that can heighten your risk of angina, but changes in the blood vessel walls also play a part. If your blood vessels remain wide open and their lining is smooth, blood flow within them remains fast and adequate. If they become narrowed, then the flow through them slows down. The change can be dramatic. Halve the diameter of a blood vessel and the flow of blood through it decreases by nine-tenths! That may still provide enough oxygen and glucose for a heart at rest, but not when you are running or even walking briskly, or climbing stairs.

I have already mentioned one cause of narrowing of these blood vessels – atheroma. However, an artery's diameter is also governed by the tone in the muscles in its walls. Every artery has in its walls muscles that encircle it. When they contract, the artery narrows, and blood flow through it slows: when they relax, the artery opens up, and the flow increases. If your arteries are in a state of constantly heightened 'tone', so that they are narrower than they should be, the blood flow through them is either less, or the pressure to keep the flow normal must rise. In the first instance, the supply of oxygen from that artery is diminished, and in the second, the demand on the heart is increased. Often, both occur together. Obviously, this is yet another set of circumstances that can promote angina.

The combination of a high level of fibrinogen, stiffened red cells, high cholesterol, high blood pressure, hyperactive aggregated platelets, and increased arterial muscle tone, all on top of atheroma in the coronary arteries, is a lethal one. Each element of that combination contributes either to lowering the supply of oxygen and glucose to the heart muscle or to increasing the demand of the heart for oxygen, and therefore to the onset of angina.

The effect of smoking on the heart

You may think that someone with all, or even some, of these angina-causing abnormalities must be very unlucky, and that they do not relate to you. Yet if you are a smoker, you possess *all* of them!

When you smoke a cigarette – and one a day is enough to show a difference – you inhale carbon monoxide, tars and nicotine. The carbon monoxide lowers the oxygen content of the blood and directly poisons the heart muscle, so that it reduces supply and makes the heart less efficient in its pumping action. The tars line the delicate tissues of the lungs, so that less oxygen can get across from the lungs into the blood – another way in which smoking reduces the supply side of the equation.

By irritating the lungs, the tars from cigarettes induce chronic inflammation and irritation, eventually leading to chronic bronchitis and emphysema. This, too, reduces the supply of oxygen to the heart. All smokers develop some degree of chronic bronchitis.

The nicotine is just as harmful. Nicotine is a powerful 'vasocon-strictor' drug, in that it stimulates the muscles around the arteries to contract, narrowing them. This is not fanciful. Volunteers who had not had a cigarette for 12 hours underwent a simple test. They allowed a tiny piece of skin to be taken from their ear lobe, and a microscope cinecamera to be focused on the blood vessel just below this place on their ear. They were then asked to inhale, once, from a cigarette. Within less than a minute, the blood vessels *in* the ear quickly contracted to half their original size or less.

Transfer that reaction to the coronary arteries. Regular smoking has a devastating effect on the flow of blood through them – more than enough to explain most attacks of angina in many people.

If that were not bad enough, smoking activates platelets, so that they clump together and start the process of thrombosis. That is further aided and abetted by the fact that smoking also raises the level of the pro-clotting factor fibrinogen in the blood, which makes clots in the coronary arteries much more probable. That can lead to heart attacks, as well as angina.

Smoking and Buerger's disease

The most extreme example of reaction to smoking is Buerger's disease, in which the blood vessels, both arteries and veins, react to tobacco by becoming extremely inflamed. The result is that their walls become much thicker than normal, and the channel through which the blood is meant to flow just 'silts up'.

If patients continue to smoke, the consequences of Buerger's disease are disastrous. They get excruciating pain in their legs, even at rest, at night, and eventually face amputations of both legs. If they stop smoking, the disease can be largely reversed. Such is the grip that smoking has on people that I have known two 'Buerger's' patients who refused to stop the habit. They both eventually had above-knee amputations of both legs, and both died from heart attacks.

Angina made worse by smoking is deadly

Because smoking plays such a great part in causing angina in so many people, I have allocated it a chapter on its own. Its influence is so great, in fact, that if you have angina, are a smoker, and are not prepared to stop, you might just as well throw this book away, or give it to someone else who will benefit from it. This is because, no matter how much treatment and care you receive from elsewhere, you are beyond help. *If exacerbated by smoking*, your angina will lead to a heart attack and death, just as night follows day.

On the other hand, just look at the benefits if you stop. No more nicotine, carbon monoxide or tars. More oxygen into your bloodstream and heart. Wide open arteries through which your less viscous blood can flow freely, and without the elements inside it that promote clotting. By the one action of stopping smoking, you will have given yourself a new lease of life that far outweighs the drug and surgical therapy that your doctors can offer. In fact, it may even be all you need to do to feel well and to lose your symptoms.

4

Why me? Looking for the causes of angina

Having read this far, you may be wondering – why me? You may not smoke, or be particularly overweight: you don't drink too much, and, as far as you know, you do not have high blood pressure or a high cholesterol level. Yet you still have angina. How can this have happened?

The last chapter explained how atheroma gives rise to angina, but it does not explain why atheroma and angina are much more common in some parts of the world than others. To understand that, we have to turn to the huge, world-encompassing studies of heart disease set up from the 1950s onwards.

The evidence from Norway concerning angina and heart disease

The first clues to the causes of heart disease came from Norway. Before the Second World War, Norwegians enjoyed a very high standard of living – *and* a very high rate of angina and deaths from heart attacks. Then came the Nazi occupation.

From 1940 onwards, Norwegians no longer had tobacco. Many were forced into jobs that were physically hard. Their milk, cheese and beef were exported to Germany, and they had to rely much more on fish as a staple food. As a nation, they lost weight and their blood pressures fell. At the same time, Norwegians were under great stress. For four years, they lived constantly with such fear and anxiety as we can hardly imagine today.

What happened to the heart attack rate under such conditions? It fell – steeply! There was also an even steeper drop in the numbers of hospital patients who had thromboses (blood clots) after surgery.

By 1947, only two years after the war ended, with the return of abundant food and cigarettes, and the immense relief from stress, the heart attack rates were rising again to the pre-war levels.

However, that Norwegian 'natural experiment', which was prob-ably mirrored in countries such as the Netherlands, also occupied by the Nazis, has lessons for us today.

The first is that, even when the answers are obvious, it is almost impossible for people to accept them if it means having to adopt a completely new approach to life. It took until the 1980s for the medical profession to accept the implications of the Norwegian experience, and only then after many other studies had confirmed them. For non-medical people, the message has still not penetrated, or it is not heeded – until they are suddenly faced with the possibility of their own mortality!

The second, and more encouraging, lesson from Norway is that it takes only a short time, less then a year, for a change in lifestyle to improve our chances of avoiding a heart attack and early death from heart disease. It does not seem possible that the lifestyle change could have reversed years of atheroma, but it may have made other differences to the supply–demand equation in the workings of the heart – such as making it much less easy for clots to form within the affected arteries.

Rates of heart disease in different countries

Countries vary enormously in the proportion of their populations with coronary heart disease. In 1986, Professor Hugh Tunstall-Pedoe of Dundee compared mortality rates from coronary heart disease in men aged 40–69 years from 30 countries. Top of the list were Northern Ireland, Finland and Scotland with 600 deaths per 100,000 men of that age range per year. England and Wales were next, followed by, in the middle, the United States, Norway, Canada and Israel, with 300–400 deaths per 100,000. Countries with much lower 'scores' – around 100–200 deaths per 100,000 – were Italy, Yugoslavia, Greece, Spain, and France. Lowest of all, by far, was Japan, with a death rate of around 50 per 100,000 – less than one-tenth of the death rates of the three top countries.

The variations are not just between countries, but within them. Within lowland Scotland, coronary deaths are high in the west and low in the east – a twofold difference in populations living only 40 or so miles apart. Districts within the biggest conurbation in western

Scotland, Glasgow, vary by as much as twofold in their heart disease death rates.

Such regional and local variations in coronary disease have given the clues to its causes. One clue was given in the 1960s by the International Atherosclerosis Project, when investigators from 14 countries in North, South and Central America, the Philippines, Jamaica, South Africa and Norway collected specimens of arteries from post-mortem examinations of 22,509 people aged from 10 to 69 years.

They showed that atheroma was present in the arteries of all people, regardless of age, race and geography. It was commoner and more extensive as they aged. However, the severe form of the disease – in which there were raised plaques with roughened surfaces projecting into the bloodstream – was closely linked to death rates from heart attacks in the countries concerned. The environment was much more important than race or gender. The severity of the atheromatous changes was directly associated with average blood cholesterol levels in the various populations.

The Seven Countries Study

Around the same time, the Seven Countries study was started in the 1960s by Professor Ancel Keys of Minneapolis. More than 12,000 men from the United States, Japan, Yugoslavia, Finland, Italy, the Netherlands and Greece were followed over five years, and then ten years. In this study, too, the key influence on heart disease was the blood cholesterol level. Cholesterol levels (measured as the percentage of men with cholesterol levels above 6.5 mmol/l) were lowest in Japan, Greece and Yugoslavia, and highest in the Netherlands, the United States and Finland. In the middle was Italy. The heart disease rates exactly mirrored that pattern.

The Seven Countries Study concluded that other factors promoting heart disease, such as smoking and high blood pressure, only come into operation if the blood cholesterol level is high. In Japan, high blood pressure is very common, and cigarette consumption is very high, yet the heart disease rate is low. Finns exercise more than nationals of other countries, yet their heart attack rate is high – and linked with their very high cholesterol level.

Where did the high blood cholesterol levels come from? The

Seven Countries Study showed conclusively that it was dietary. When the blood cholesterol levels in each country were compared with the percentage of dietary calories derived from animal fats (containing saturated fatty acids), the Finns were far and away at the top of the graph, and the Japanese were at the opposite pole. There was a very close correlation between eating saturated fats and blood cholesterol levels in each country.

The North Karelia Project

The Finns were stung enough by their poor performance rates to do something about them. They started their North Karelia Project in 1972, and it is still continuing. The North Karelian Health and Social Services departments combined in an onslaught on heart disease, with the specific aim of reducing smoking, blood pressure and the amount of saturated fats (mainly red meat and dairy products) in the diet. The mass media co-operated in the Project. From 1974 to 1979, in North Karelia there was a 22 per cent reduction in coronary heart disease deaths, compared with a 12 per cent reduction in neighbouring Kuopio, and an 11 per cent reduction in Finland minus Kuopio and North Karelia. In 1982 the difference was still evident, showing that community-based programmes giving a strong health message can work. However, the message has to be continued for each generation: more recent reports, in the 1990s concerning Finland, suggest that the current population are backsliding and that their heart disease rates are rising again.

The Framingham study and the British Regional Heart Study

While the Finns were taking action, the Americans and British were still gathering data. The classic study of heart disease in individuals is that produced in the small New England community of Framingham, 18 miles west of Boston in the United States. In 1948, 5,000 men and women aged 30–59 years from the population of 28,000 were recruited into a long-term study. They were to be examined every two years, indefinitely.

They, and several more groups recruited at intervals since then, are still under study. Well over half of the original group have died, and their illnesses and causes of death have been scrutinized in detail. The British Regional Heart Study (referred to in the Introduction) started in 1978 is also continuing.

The American and British results are similar, despite their great differences in geography and lifestyles. In Framingham, in general, smokers died several years before non-smokers, from heart attacks, as well as from lung diseases such as cancer and bronchitis. Men and women with diabetes also tended to have heart and circulation disorders that shortened their lives.

What surprised the doctors in the Framingham study most, though, was the very close link between death from heart attacks and the level of blood cholesterol. A higher than average cholesterol level put the men at particularly high risk of a coronary death, the risk being multiplied many times more if it was linked with cigarette smoking, and even higher still if high blood pressure was added.

The Framingham study raised crucial questions for the American authorities. Could control of cholesterol, smoking and high blood pressure be the answer to the heart disease pandemic that was killing half the American population?

Risk factors for angina and heart disease

The British had been aware of their problem for more than a century. In 1871, a Dr Haviland alluded to big differences in the numbers of deaths from heart disease in different regions of England and Wales. To the north of a line from the Severn to the Wash, he wrote, people were especially prone to heart disease. South of the line, they seemed to be protected against it.

That line divided the prosperous south from the poorer north in Victorian Britain, but the differences were still there in 1978, the year of the start of the British Regional Heart Study. The Scottish towns had twice the heart attack rates of towns on the English south coast – and there was a gradient from low to high in the towns in between, so that each town had a higher heart attack rate than its neighbour to the south, and a lower rate than its neighbour to the north.

The British Regional Heart Study divided the subjects into risk groups – according to age, smoking habit, Body Mass Index (BMI) (a measure of obesity), blood pressure and blood cholesterol levels. It also divided them on whether they had signs of heart disease before entering the study. The results have painted a very accurate picture of who is at highest risk of angina and heart attacks, and why.

Age Over all, among the 7,735 men in the British Regional Heart Study, the heart attack rate was 6.2 per 1,000 men per year. The rate was 2/1,000/year for the 40–44-year-olds, gradually rising to 10/1,000/year in the 55–59-year-olds. Forty per cent of the cases were fatal, and about half of the deaths happened within an hour of the start of the chest pain. These results were a major stimulus to today's coronary care service, about which more later. Suffice it to say that many lives are now saved by the emergency ambulance service paramedics who aim to reach every reported chest pain within 15 minutes with full emergency equipment on board.

Smoking Although ex-smokers in the British Regional Heart Study still retained twice the risk of a heart attack than a 'never smoker', stopping did reduce the chances of an attack. Smokers were at much higher risk of a heart attack than non-smokers and ex-smokers.

Body Mass Index (BMI) Body Mass Index is a convenient way of measuring how your weight relates to your height – in other words, it tells you if you are too fat, too thin or just right! The formula sounds complicated, but it is easy to work out if you know your height in metres and your weight in kilograms. Figure 3 shows how it works.

BMI is the weight in kilograms divided by the square of the height in metres. If you know your height in inches, multiply that by 2.54 for centimetres and divide by 100. This gives you your height in metres. Likewise, if you know your weight in pounds, multiply that by 0.4536 to give you your weight in kilograms. Take as an example a man of 5 feet 10 inches and who weighs 12 stones 9 pounds. Therefore he is 70 inches (1.778 metres) tall, and weighs 177 pounds (approximately 80 kilograms). The square of his height (i.e. 1.778 x 1.778) equals 3.16. Now divide 80 (his weight) by the square (3.16) and the answer is 25.3.

This figure of 25.3 is the man's BMI. It is just at the upper limit of normal, so shows that he is just a pound or two overweight. However, a BMI of 27 or more could be considered overweight enough to do something about it, and a BMI of 30-plus is obese.

It is generally considered that a BMI range of 20–25 is within normal limits: below 20 is probably too thin, and above 27 too fat. In the British Regional Heart Study, men above the average of 20–25 for BMI were at higher risk than average of having a heart attack.

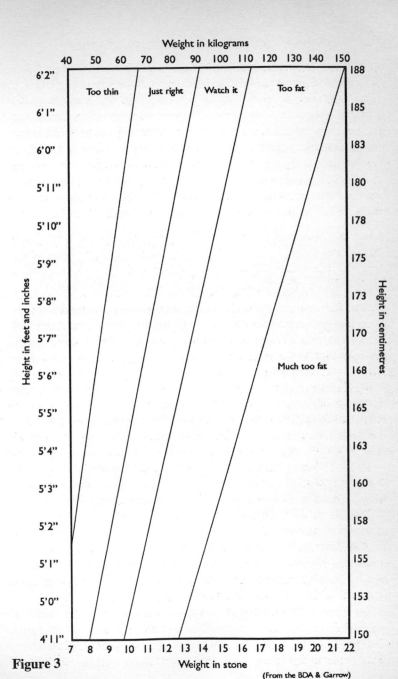

Figure 3

(From the BDA & Garrow)

However, a high BMI is closely related to a high cholesterol level, to high blood pressure and to another measure of fats in the blood, a high triglyceride level. When these were taken into account in the British Regional Heart Study analysis, the BMI alone did not appear to exert an extra effect on heart disease over and above them. Some people have taken this to mean that obesity does not really matter, as long as you keep your blood pressure and blood fat levels under control. This is not true, and in any case is very difficult to achieve, as obesity, fat and blood pressure are all bound up together. So if you are overweight and have angina, it is best to lose the extra weight.

Blood pressure A blood pressure measurement has two readings – the 'systolic' and the 'diastolic' pressures. Systole is the contraction of the heart which pumps the blood into the main arteries, and diastole is the relaxation phase, in which the heart fills up again with blood entering from the veins and the lungs. During diastole, valves close to stop the blood in the arteries rushing back into the heart, and the arteries tense, exerting a further pressure on the blood inside them, so that it continues on its way.

Pressures are measured in millimetres of mercury (mm Hg). The systolic pressure is the pressure exerted on the blood in systole, the normal being around 120–140 mm Hg, and the diastolic pressure, measured during diastole, is around 70–90 mm Hg. Blood pressures are noted down as the systolic/diastolic reading, such as 125/80 mm Hg.

As blood pressure rises, so does the risk of a heart attack. The British Regional Heart Study revealed that at a systolic pressure equal to or higher than 148 mm Hg, the heart attack risk was twice normal. There was a raised risk too if the resting diastolic pressure was, on repeated measuring, above 93 mm Hg, but even those with diastolic pressures above 72 mm Hg appeared to carry some extra risk. This result was similar to those in American studies, which suggest that the lower the diastolic blood pressure, the better it is for the heart.

Cholesterol Cholesterol, of course, was the big story of the 1980s. As in the Framingham study, the British Regional Heart Study found that the higher the blood cholesterol level, the greater the heart attack risk. Those in the top fifth for cholesterol (7.2 mmol/l or more) had three times the heart attacks of those in the bottom fifth (less than 5.5 mmol/l). However, there were some heart attacks in those with a relatively low cholesterol level, suggesting that there is no level of blood cholesterol (in Britain, at least) at which there is no heart attack risk. This is perhaps not surprising, as even the lowest levels of cholesterol here would be considered very high in, say, China, where a blood cholesterol level above 4 mmol/l is very unusual. Perhaps in Britain we *all* have too high a cholesterol level.

Here we should bring in the views of Professor Michael Oliver, now retired, but whose main career was spent in the University of Edinburgh's Cardiovascular Research Unit. He worked for years on the reasons for Scotland's unenviable position as the country with the most 'heart' deaths. He points out that the southern French smoke as much as the Scots, eat as much fat as the Scots, and have high cholesterol levels – yet they have far less trouble with angina and fewer heart attacks.

Professor Oliver is convinced that it is not the amount of cholesterol in the blood that determines the heart attack risk, but the quality of that fat. He then compared the heart attack rates of Scots, Finns, Swedes (who have a low heart attack rate) and southern Italians (with an even lower heart attack rate than the Swedes).

Crucial to the heart attack rate in these four populations was the level of linoleic acid in the blood. The *higher* the linoleic acid level, the *lower* was the heart attack risk. The levels were negligible in the Scots and high in the Italians and Swedes.

Linoleic acid is a polyunsaturated fat, found in cereals and some vegetable oils such as olive oil – which is heavily used in cooking by the Italians and other Mediterranean countries. Linked with the linoleic acid intake is what has been called the 'Mediterranean diet', with its reliance on fish, citrus fruits, garlic, green vegetables – all substances, according to Professor Oliver, that help prevent the blood clotting that is the first step towards a heart attack. Not surprisingly, Professor Oliver endorses a Mediterranean-style of eating for everyone, and especially for those who already have evidence of heart disease.

Interestingly, he also directly links smoking with high blood cholesterol and linoleic acid levels. His team's research showed that coronary-prone people, such as people with angina or who have already had heart attacks, do not eat much food that contains linoleic acid. Smokers were even more selective about their choice of food: they had real dislikes for foods containing the 'protective' fats. The more cigarettes they smoked, the less linoleic acid they had in their tissues. They ate less fish and less vegetable fibre than non-smokers. The difference also applied to alcohol consumption: smokers drank more than non-smokers.

Professor Oliver postulated that smoking injures the taste buds, so that food containing protective fats and oils tastes less pleasant, so that it is rejected, perhaps subconsciously. Smokers also add more than the normal amount of salt to their food, a habit that tends to suggest that smoking changes – or, to be more accurate, poisons – the ability to taste.

Pre-existing heart disease A crucial group within the British Regional Heart Study were those who already had signs of heart disease when they were first enrolled in the survey in 1978. Doctors tended to believe at that time that once a heart attack had occurred, there was little point in trying to reduce the risks by altering lifestyle, because the damage to the heart was already done, and could not be undone or reversed.

The Study showed, on the contrary, that the risk factors still mattered. Even after a heart attack, those with higher cholesterol and blood pressure levels were at higher risk than their colleagues in whom they were lower. It was concluded from this that even after an attack it was wise to keep the risks as low as possible, by whatever means possible.

No risk factor – no heart attack? It is often said, mostly by those who do not wish to change their own lives, that many heart attack victims do not have any identifiable risk factors, such as smoking, a high blood cholesterol level or high blood pressure. However, the British Regional Heart Study gave the lie to that.

In the Study, men with either:

- a serum cholesterol level equal to or above 6.0 mmol/l
- a systolic blood pressure equal to or above 148 mm Hg

- a diastolic blood pressure equal to or above 93 mm Hg

or who:

- currently smoked cigarettes

had twice the risk of a heart attack than the others.

Only 5 of the 202 cases of major heart attack in the British Regional Heart Study did not meet one of these criteria, and over two-thirds of them met at least two of them. Of the five men not meeting the criteria, three had evidence of a previous heart attack.

So only one in a hundred of the cases of heart attack possessed none of the risk factors listed, and this does not take into account previous smoking habit, treatment for high blood pressure, or a change in eating habits that might have lowered serum cholesterol. We can let Professor Shaper, the author of the Study, have the last word on it. He wrote in his booklet entitled *Coronary Heart Disease: Risks and Reasons* (1988, Current Medical Literature Ltd): 'It would appear that major coronary heart disease events virtually do not occur in middle aged British men in the absence of at least one significantly increased risk factor.'

I would add two corollaries to that statement. The first is that it surely applies to women as well. The second is that if anyone with angina wishes to avoid a heart attack, and at the same time improve his or her angina, then the best way to go about it must surely be to lose any current risk factor. The next chapters show you exactly how to do that.

5

Reducing the risk factors –
tackling cholesterol: the evidence

The previous chapters strongly suggest that the main problem for people with angina is fat – cholesterol – in the bloodstream and arteries. If that can be reduced, then the risk of the angina getting worse or leading to a heart attack should be reduced. The problem, though, is how to do it.

The Norwegian experience alluded to in Chapter 4 offers some evidence that eating differently may help, although so many aspects of life changed in Norway during the Nazi occupation that the effect of any one of them alone cannot be judged. The fact that the heart attack rate responded so rapidly to the changed circumstances (within a year) strongly suggests that it was a change in thrombosis rates, rather than any improvement in atheroma in the coronary artery walls, that made the difference.

Does reducing cholesterol reduce the risk of angina and heart disease?

Can atheroma actually be reversed, once established in an artery? Professor R.W. Wissler of Chicago showed that atheroma in monkeys and pigs can be made to regress towards normality after one to four years of a low-fat diet. Their blood cholesterol levels became normal, the plaques became smaller, and the plaques themselves contained less cholesterol. There was less risk of thrombosis on the surface of the plaques, many of which healed over, so that the arterial inner surface was much smoother. Professor Wissler's findings appear in *A Textbook of Cardiovascular Medicine* (Edited by E. Braunwald, 1984, W. B. Saunders, Chicago).

The implication of the animal work is that a similar reduction in dietary fats in people should improve angina and help prevent heart attacks. But does it? It has been difficult for researchers to produce hard evidence that it does.

Since the 1950s there have been many large trials to determine whether reducing blood cholesterol levels will improve coronary heart disease and prevent heart attacks. They have used diet and drugs, mostly in middle-aged men, and their results have been mixed. Perhaps this is because it is over-optimistic to expect that a small change in blood cholesterol levels will improve, in a short time, a disease that has been present for many years (usually since childhood).

What is cholesterol?

Before going into these trials, however, a few facts about cholesterol would not go amiss. We have all been bombarded by the food industry and health pundits with the need to reduce cholesterol levels, but how many people really understand what it is? My guess is very few.

It is normal to have cholesterol in the bloodstream. It is a fatty substance used by the body to maintain organs such as the liver and brain, the structure of the cells of which is fat-based. It is a 'building brick' for complex steroid hormones such as cortisone and sex hormones.

Therefore we cannot do without cholesterol. However, we do need to keep its levels in the blood within certain limits. If it is too high, the excess appears to be deposited in the walls of the blood vessels, along with other fats (lipids). This produces first the fatty streaks, then the atheromatous plaques, mentioned in Chapter 3.

How high a cholesterol level is too high?

This has been determined internationally by authorities such as the US National Heart Lung and Blood Institute, the Study Group of the European Atherosclerosis Society, and the World Health Organisation MONICA Project (MONitoring trends In CArdiovascular disease).

Via a simple blood test, cholesterol levels are measured in millimols per litre (mmol/l) in Europe, or in milligrams per decilitre (mg/dl) in the United States. 1 mmol/l equals 38.6 mg/dl, so that total blood cholesterol levels of 6.0 mmol/l and 240 mg/dl are the same.

The experts have agreed that cholesterol levels are becoming moderately high when they are above 5.2 mmol/l, and need definite attention when they rise above 6.5 mmol/l. People are defined as

41

'hyperlipidaemic' (a serious high blood-fat level needing medical treatment) if their blood cholesterol is above 7.8 mmol/l. Doctors try to keep patients in a range between 4 to 5 mmol/l.

That sounds fairly simple, but the reality is different. To begin with, even average levels of cholesterol in developed countries are well above 5.2 mmol/l. In 1989, Dr Hugh Tunstall-Pedoe and his colleagues in Dundee measured blood cholesterol levels in more than 10,000 men and women aged between 25 and 64. Three-quarters of them had cholesterol levels above 5.2: a third had levels over 6.5, and in one-tenth they were above 7.8! Dr Tunstall-Pedoe drew two main conclusions from his study. The first was that it confirmed why we Scots are so unhealthy, and have such a high rate of angina and heart attack. He added, however, that the figures are not so different from anywhere else in Europe. The second was that so many people have high blood cholesterol levels that advice on how to lower them could be given to everyone, without the need to spend time and money testing for it.

This view was contested for a while, when reports appeared that too low a cholesterol level might be just as harmful as an excess. Dr Christopher Isles, studying cholesterol levels in 15,000 men and women in Renfrew and Paisley, towns just to the west of Glasgow, found that the people with the lowest cholesterol levels (below 4 mmol/l) were more likely than the others to die from cancer. In his study, the people with the lowest death rates over all had cholesterol levels of around 5.6 mmol/l.

These figures suggested that it would be wrong to advise the whole population to lower their cholesterol level. However, follow-up research since then has shown that the cancer occurring in patients with a very low level of cholesterol may in fact have pre-dated the measurement of their cholesterol. The cancer may have exhausted the body's cholesterol-forming mechanism, and the fall in their cholesterol levels may have been *due* to their illness and not vice versa. It is now accepted that lowering cholesterol from around 6 mmol/l to around 4 mmol/l (the aim of most dietary regimens) does not increase the risk of any illness, but substantially reduces angina and heart attack rates.

The same goes for another curious link with lowered cholesterol. Several early studies suggested that although lowering cholesterol reduced heart attack deaths, it was linked with increased deaths from accident, suicide and violence. These have turned out to be statistical eccentricities, and not true differences. It is difficult to see how reducing blood cholesterol levels could make a person more vulnerable to a mugger's attack or to death from a road accident!

Does lowering cholesterol actually improve heart disease? Dozens of studies have set out to answer this question, but few have given adequate answers. This is mainly because of flaws in the design of the trials, rather than that cholesterol reduction was in fact a failure. The first few trials of cholesterol reduction were aimed at whole populations, without screening for cholesterol levels.

The 'whole population' approach to reducing cholesterol

Among the early studies was the Los Angeles Veterans Administration Study, which took place between 1959 and 1967. This followed 846 men aged between 54 and 88 years, of whom a quarter initially had evidence of coronary heart disease (mainly angina). Half were allocated to a diet in which the ratio of polyunsaturated fats to saturated fats was 2:1 – vegetable and fish oils were used instead of animal fats. Half were left as 'controls'. After eight years, fewer deaths from heart disease and non-fatal heart attacks had occurred in the 'treatment' group (85 in 424) than in the 'controls' (119 in 422). The benefit of cholesterol lowering was greatest in the men under 65 years old.

Diet also seemed to work in 700 men and 600 women in the Finnish Mental Hospitals Study, which was undertaken from 1959 to 1971. For six years, those in one hospital were on the same polyunsaturated/saturated 2:1 diet as in the Los Angeles study, whereas those in the other hospital were left alone. After six years, the positions were reversed. Although the patient populations changed greatly during the 12 years, and there were many problems with the data analysis, the diet was linked with a moderate benefit in reduction of heart attack and stroke for both men and women (though less so for women).

The North Karelia Study described in Chapter 4, which targeted a whole community, produced a similar benefit, in that heart attacks became fewer after the 'low cholesterol' educational project started.

Factory-based health education

However, not all educational projects have succeeded like the Finnish one. The WHO (World Health Organisation) European Collaborative Trial was an attempt to prevent coronary heart disease using factory-based health education. The subjects were 49,781 men aged 40–59 years, working in 44 pairs of factories in Britain, Belgium, Italy, Spain and Poland. The health education message was given to everyone working at the 'treatment' factories, and not to those in the 'control' factories.

Over all, after six years, there was an average reduction in coronary heart disease *risk* of 11 per cent, and an average reduction of 8 per cent in actual *deaths* from coronary disease, in the 'treatment' factories compared to the 'control' factories. However, the different countries varied in their success rates. The best successes were in Italy and Belgium, and in Britain there was no benefit at all, except in that by the end of the study fewer men were smoking.

The Belgian results were particularly interesting, in that the men in the 'treatment' factories with angina and an abnormal ECG at the start of the study showed the greatest proportionate decrease in heart attacks. In the 'control' factories, the heart attack rates in such men were 138 per 1,000 men: in the 'treatment' factories, they were 63 per 1,000. This meant that the health education message was halving the heart attack rate in the men at highest risk – and this should be an encouragement to any reader with angina.

Why were the Belgians so different from the British? It is hardly likely that they are genetically different. Are British factory workers less likely to listen to a health message than their Belgian colleagues, or was the message not put across in a satisfactory way by the researchers in Britain? The answer is unclear, but one message from that trial was that a considerable effort is needed to make major changes in a society.

The 'high-risk' approach to reducing cholesterol

Another approach to the cholesterol problem was to target only those with high blood cholesterol levels, and to treat them with drugs. Drugs to lower blood cholesterol levels were studied first in the 1970s, but they have had a troubled history since then.

WHO and clofibrate

The first study, the WHO Cooperative Trial of the drug clofibrate, followed 15,745 healthy men in Edinburgh, Budapest and Prague. Treatment was based on their cholesterol levels. Those in the upper third for blood cholesterol levels were allocated at random either to the cholesterol-lowering drug clofibrate, or to a placebo. Those in the lower third for cholesterol levels were also given a placebo – they were the 'baseline' control. The study was double blind, so that researchers and patients did not know what they were taking or in what group they were.

The results for heart attacks were mildly encouraging, as the clofibrate group had fewer non-fatal heart attacks than the high-cholesterol group given a placebo. However, the clofibrate group had the highest overall number of deaths – a result that stopped the use of the drug in its tracks! This was despite its lowering the cholesterol levels by an average of 9 per cent.

The excess of deaths of people taking clofibrate were not due to a single disease or discernible cause. The greatest benefit of cholesterol lowering was in younger men with moderately raised cholesterol levels, but this was overshadowed by the unexpected extra deaths. The use of cholesterol-lowering drugs in anyone other than people with extremely high cholesterol levels has never fully recovered from that trial result.

The Multiple Risk Factor Intervention Trial (MRFIT)

MRFIT was an American study of 361,662 men aged 35–57 who volunteered for health screening through their employment. Some 12,866 in the upper range for risk, based on smoking, blood pressure and blood cholesterol level, and who showed no evidence of heart disease, were admitted to the trial.

Half the group (6,428 men) were allocated to a programme of special intervention. They were seen every four months, asked to stop smoking, had their blood pressure well controlled, and asked to alter their eating habits to reduce their blood cholesterol. The other half (6,438 men) were given 'usual care', which meant that they were seen once a year and given no specific advice about how to change their coronary risks. However, they and their doctors were given all necessary information about their risk factors.

The 'control' group, however, still got the health message, because smoking, blood pressure and blood cholesterol levels were reduced in both groups – though significantly more so in the 'treatment' group.

Over seven years, the heart attack morality was 22 per cent less in the treatment group than in the control group. This difference, however, did not meet the criteria for statistical significance, partly because heart attack rates in the controls also fell, to almost half the rate expected from the Framingham experience. More detailed analysis suggested that the main causes of the reduction in problems for both groups were stopping smoking and reduction of cholesterol levels.

The Oslo Study Group

Norwegians, like Scots, feature highly in studies of heart disease. The Oslo Study Group screened 16,202 men aged 40–49 years for coronary risk factors. They then selected 1,232 healthy men at high risk (because of smoking and high cholesterol levels) to see whether lowering serum cholesterol and stopping smoking would reduce their heart attack rate. The men had initial blood cholesterol levels of 7.5–9.8 mmol/l and 80 per cent of them smoked cigarettes. Half were given health advice (the 'treatment' group), and half (the 'control' group) were not.

After five years, the cholesterol levels were 13 per cent lower, and the number of cigarettes smoked each day 45 per cent lower, in the 'treatment' group than in the 'control' group. These were linked with a 47 per cent reduction in fatal and non-fatal heart attacks in the 'treatment' group. The statistics were clear: there were 22 non-fatal heart attacks per 1,000 men over the five years in the 'treatment' group, and 35 in the controls. The corresponding figures for deaths were 26 and 38.

Detailed analysis of the Oslo study suggested that the improvement in the rate for heart attacks and deaths were mainly due to cholesterol lowering, and less linked with stopping smoking.

The Lipid Research Clinics Study

In this American study, 480,000 men aged 35–59 were screened, yielding 18,000 with blood cholesterol levels of at least 6.85 mmol/l. For four months, these 18,000 men were asked to stick to a cholesterol-lowering diet. The 80 per cent who did so successfully, and brought their cholesterol down to normal levels, were then asked to continue on their diet. The rest of the trial concentrated on the 20 per cent (3,806 men) who were then given drug 'treatment', or a placebo (the 'control' group).

The drug used was cholestyramine, which has a different action from clofibrate. After seven years, the drug-treated group had blood cholesterol levels 9 per cent lower than the controls; they had a 19 per cent lower rate of fatal and non-fatal heart attacks; there were 20 per cent fewer cases of angina: and they needed 21 per cent fewer coronary bypass operations.

Although the figures are encouraging, the differences between the two groups are small, and perhaps not enough to encourage the use of cholestyramine generally.

These findings have, however, created enthusiasm for treating 'high-risk' (i.e. high blood cholesterol) angina patients with cholestyramine, and certainly for vigorously promoting a diet for them that would lower their cholesterol levels. Whether there would be much benefit in promoting the treatment for men with lower blood cholesterol levels remains in doubt.

The London Civil Servant Study

Lowering a particular population's cholesterol level by advice on health alone can be done, if it is approached with enthusiasm. In a study of London civil servants aged 40–49 years, half were given simple dietary recommendations aimed at lowering blood cholesterol. Over only four months, the average blood cholesterol level fell by 10 per cent, but – more importantly – the percentage of men with a blood cholesterol over 6.2 mmol/l changed from 53 per cent to 25 per cent. After 18 months, only 23 per cent of them had blood cholesterol figures above 6.2 mmol/l.

This must have greatly reduced their potential for a premature heart attack. When the cholesterol levels were divided up into five equal blocks from the lowest to the highest, it turned out that only 7 per cent of the heart attacks occurred in people in the lower two-fifths. Thirty-one per cent of the heart attacks occurred in the top one-fifth for cholesterol level. This is a strong argument for lowering a high cholesterol level into the normal range by changing our lifestyles.

47

Summarizing the trials

All the trials aiming to reduce the heart attack rate by lowering cholesterol levels have met with some success, but in most the success has been less spectacular than expected. The limitations have been partly caused by the design of the trials – the 'control' groups have often taken to healthier lifestyles as the news of the good effects started to spread.

A main problem with the cholesterol-lowering trials, however, has been their concentration on cholesterol only, and not on all the circumstances that contribute to heart attacks, such as high blood pressure, obesity, lack of exercise, smoking and alcohol. In any doctor/patient discussion, all the risks would be put before the patient, and then doctor and patient would work together to reduce or abolish them. This was deliberately not done in many of the trials, as their aim was specifically to measure the effect of cholesterol lowering.

The Veritas Society and the doctors who don't believe that raised cholesterol is dangerous

This chapter would not be complete if it did not mention the doctors who disagree with the whole cholesterol story. They have banded together to form the Veritas Society, a leading light of which is George V. Mann, an American nutritionist and doctor who was an associate director of the Framingham study for three years. The Veritas Society exists to fight the hypothesis that the fat content of food determines the level of cholesterol in the blood and the risk of coronary heart disease.

Its members met in Washington DC on 13 November 1991, and their deliberations were published in *Coronary Heart Disease, the Dietary Sense and Nonsense* George V. Mann (1993, Janus Publishing Company). The gist of the book is that the American food and drugs manufacturing companies have conspired together to construct a scare around blood cholesterol levels for their own profit, and the US authorities and public have been taken in by them.

Dr Mann puts the blame for the current high rate of angina on 'trans' fatty acids, which are mainly non-natural fats that occur during the manufacture of margarines from seed oils. He listed common foods in the United States that contain very high levels of trans fatty acids, such as biscuits, sweets, French fries, puddings, pastries, crisps and, of course, margarine. For Dr Mann, animal fats and butter are much healthier than manufactured margarines and many manufactured 'low saturated fat' foods.

He goes further, citing the mortality rates for female vegetarians as evidence for his theory. Female vegetarians, he says, have a higher death rate from heart disease than female non-vegetarians; and a very much higher death rate from all causes. The differences do not apply to males. Dr Mann does not give an exact definition of 'vegetarian', and without further supporting evidence his claims cannot be considered conclusive.

I do not know for sure whether Dr Mann is correct, or whether he and his colleagues in the Veritas Society are just maverick eccentrics, outside the mainstream of informed opinion. However, even if his views are eventually found to be correct, it would not make much difference to the advice I would give to most people with angina. This is because living with angina is not just a question of cholesterol and diet: it is a matter of changing your life in many ways, not just the fat content of your food.

My own feeling is that all the trials point towards the same conclusion: that changing our lifestyles (by stopping smoking, losing weight, eating differently and exercising more) can help us to avoid or diminish angina and prevent a heart attack. In future, new drugs may help further, but the onus will always be on ourselves to do the best we can – and how we can do it is described later.

6

Reducing the risk factors –
your changing lifestyle

Having read this far, you should now be convinced that you will
benefit from losing your 'risk factors' – although you may not be
convinced that you *can* do it!

You have two obvious ways to reverse the process that is causing
your angina. First, you can reduce the work done by your heart –
thereby lessening the demand for oxygen and glucose – and secondly,
you can improve the circulation in your coronary arteries so that they
can deliver a better supply of oxygen and glucose. If you can do both
together, so much the better.

There are three more, less obvious, options. First, you can make
the blood flowing through the coronary arteries carry more oxygen;
and secondly, you can make the blood less viscous, so that it flows
more easily. Third, you can help to make the heart muscle work more
efficiently, so that it needs less oxygen to do the same amount of
work. We will touch on all these options in this chapter.

The first step

The first step is to get into a routine with your angina. Whenever the
pain starts, wherever you are, you must stop and rest completely, and
remain at rest for 30 minutes. This gives your heart time to recover
from the 'ischaemic' episode. Note the attack down, how severe it
was, its relationship to exercise or exertion, how long it took to
subside, and how soon you restarted your activities.

From then on, your aim is to try, week by week, to improve your
tolerance of exercise. Keep on exercising: both walking and
swimming are good exercises that will improve the efficiency of your
heart, but remember always to stop at the first sign of discomfort.
Keep writing your notes, and you will find that you can improve the
distances you walked, or the slopes you can tackle, or the time for
which you can exercise. That can be a big boost to your confidence,
and will encourage you to continue.

Avoiding cigarette smoke

Your heart's efficacy will improve if you can keep your coronary arteries as wide open as possible. Crucial to that aim is to avoid cigarette smoke – your own and other people's. Exposure to cigarette smoke narrows all the small arteries in the skin, pushing up the blood pressure, and causing the coronary arteries to shut down. If they are already narrowed as a result of atheroma, then narrowing them further at the same time as increasing the work of the heart is both insane and suicidal.

Stopping smoking completely is essential: it is no use 'cutting down' or 'trying to stop'. The *only* answer, if you are a smoker, is to say to yourself that you are, from this moment on, a non-smoker. If you can't do that, then it does not matter how good you are at taking the rest of the advice – you are lost.

Keeping away from other people's smoke is vital too. Despite the claims of the tobacco companies to the contrary, there is plenty of evidence that other people's smoking gets nicotine into the bloodstream of non-smokers. Nicotine breaks down in the body to a poisonous substance called cotinine, and non-smokers who work in smoky atmospheres have measurable levels of cotinine in their blood. The more their colleagues or customers smoke, the higher their own blood cotinine levels are. The same applies to your home. The babies of parents who smoke have cotinine in their blood; and the higher the level, the more likely they are to be admitted to hospital with lung disease. For every 20 cigarettes smoked around them, non-smokers passively smoke the equivalent of one cigarette.

So if you have angina, avoid cigarette smoke at all costs. In today's social climate, we should not feel embarrassed to ask smokers nearby to stop smoking, or to go elsewhere to do so. In your home, a small, discreet non-smoking sign on the window can deter visitors from lighting up, but if they know you have angina, then a quiet word of explanation why they should not smoke in the house should be perfectly acceptable.

Eating better

At the same time, start on your long-term plan to reverse your angina. We do not yet have the hard proof that human beings can reverse already established atheromatous plaques in their arteries by changing their lifestyles, but it seems reasonable to infer, from all the evidence of animal and human volunteer studies, that we can. And there is good evidence, from angiogram studies, that a better lifestyle can prevent the development of new plaques.

The best way to change is to convert to an eating pattern that you really like, and can enthuse about for the rest of your life. That is not so difficult as it seems, for the 'Mediterranean' style of eating espoused by Professor Oliver (described in Chapter 4) is delicious, as well as healthy and relatively cheap!

The main aim of the new life you must lead is to lower your blood cholesterol level. Cholesterol reaches the bloodstream from two sources: in our food (as in eggs or liver), and from our own livers, which make cholesterol from the fats (mainly animal fats) eaten in food. The cholesterol we consume in eggs and liver is much less important than animal fats as a source of our blood cholesterol, so that we can eat two to three eggs a week or liver once a week, if we like these foods, without worry. Labelling foods as 'cholesterol-free' is just a gimmick.

What really seems to matter is how much fat we eat, and the proportion of it that is derived from animals, rather than fish or vegetables. We get most of our fats from red meat and dairy products, such as cream, cheese, butter and full-cream milk. The official recommendation is that fats should only account for between 30 and 35 per cent of the total calorie intake in our food. This is well below the content of animal fats in most British diets.

This is especially true for children. For most British children, 40 per cent of their food energy supply comes from animal fats: this rises to 50 per cent or more for children reared on 'junk' foods. This is potentially tragic, because atheroma starts in childhood, and hamburgers and chips are the best way to raise cholesterol levels in children.

Yet there is no need to be a food faddist, or to avoid one sort of food altogether. Even if you have angina, you can enjoy a wide variety of foods. There are simple rules you should observe, though. The first is to grill foods, or fry them in vegetable oils rather than fats or butter. Very small children may need some full-cream milk for extra energy, but for most of us it is better to drink or cook with semi-skimmed or skimmed milk rather than whole milk.

For the most part, butter and hard margarines should be replaced by low-fat soft spreads made from buttermilk or skimmed milk, or by soft margarines made from polyunsaturated vegetable oils. Choose cheeses that have a low fat content, such as cottage cheese, rather than traditional hard or high-fat cheeses.

Use vegetable oils for cooking, and eat more fish, poultry and vegetables than red meats. There is no need to cut out beef, lamb and pork altogether, but it may be wise to restrict them to twice a week.

Here I would like to plug (yet again) the 'Mediterranean' way of eating. The ideal is to 'go Italian'! Italian food is not only among the best in the world, but it is among the healthiest too! Italians cook mainly in olive oil, eat plenty of high-quality vegetables and fruit, their fish is superb, and they eat meat sparingly.

Pasta is starchy rather than sugary, so that your glucose level rises slowly after a meal, if at all (starch takes longer to digest down to glucose than does sugar). That is all to the good. Even the garlic used in Italian cooking helps. Garlic contains substances that help to prevent the blood clotting. Eating garlic every day may not make you popular with close friends (unless they are eating it too!), but it may help you live longer.

The most important aspect of this change of eating habit (I deliberately do not call it a 'diet') is that it is a positive one. It is not a question of cutting down on food intake, but of shifting to a more varied, tastier and healthier way of eating. You can be just as satisfied after an Italian meal than after the 'meat and two veg' so beloved of the British.

The new tastes you encounter on the way to your new style of living will be a revelation. Experiment with spices, and use less salt, so that you can taste these new flavours. As desire for salt diminishes, your sensitivity to other tastes will be enhanced – *and* you will not put on weight.

Not everyone wants to eat Italian-style all the time, though. There are alternatives, such as a baked potato instead of pasta, or onions instead of garlic. Now that you have made fish and poultry your main source of protein, grill them or shallow fry them in oil. For extra taste and interest, try frying them in oatmeal. However, do not use the cooking oil more than three times: repeated frying can turn unsaturated oils into saturated fats.

Do not forget the vegetables and fruit. In the last 20 years there has been a huge expansion in the variety of vegetables and fruits in British shops. We are no longer limited to seasonal vegetables, such as cabbages, brussels sprouts, carrots and peas. We can now buy broccoli, courgettes, peppers, aubergines, avocados and dozens of other vegetables all year round.

The same goes for fruits. Oranges come in all shapes, sizes and degrees of sweetness, and we can buy fresh pineapple, grapes, melons, kiwi fruits, pawpaws, mangoes and guavas. As with vegetables, we are no longer limited to seasonal fruits such as apples, plums and pears.

The rule is to eat at least five portions of fruit and of vegetables every day. They are not only enjoyable, but they can be a positive aid to improving the circulation. Recent research suggests that 'anti-oxidant' substances, which are found in abundance in fruit, vegetables and cereals (anti-oxidants include vitamins C and E), are vital to the health and integrity of the arterial walls. They may even help to reverse the changes of atheroma, so tuck in to them!

Changing your style of eating will do more than just reduce your cholesterol levels: it may also improve your circulation, and will, in any case, be very pleasant and fulfilling.

Losing weight

I wrote about Body Mass Index (BMI) in Chapter 4. If you are overweight (with a BMI above 27) and have angina, it is best to lose enough weight to return to the 20–25 BMI range.

One reason for losing weight is that your heart then has less work to do at rest and during exercise, so the demand for blood flow through your coronary arteries falls. Even if that drop in demand is slight, every little improvement in the supply–demand equation counts. Fat people are more likely to have angina and a heart attack than thin people, but the relationship is not straightforward. Many thin people also have heart attacks.

Nevertheless, it is better to be of normal weight than to be overweight, even if obesity of itself is not a direct cause of coronary disease. If you are overweight, you are likely to have a higher blood cholesterol level than normal, and your blood pressure is likely to be raised too. In the process of losing weight, you may also return both cholesterol and blood pressure to normal. You will also feel better, and be happier about the way you look. Being at ease with your looks can help to relieve underlying anxieties, which in themselves are an extra demand on the heart.

How should you lose weight? There are only three choices open to you. You must exercise more, or eat less, or do both. If your angina is severe, then you must exercise under supervision at first, to the best of your ability, but try to gauge it to a level just below that which brings on angina. Eating less is more difficult for people who have eaten well all their lives. Perhaps the most important advice on eating is to forget about the social convention that we should eat three meals a day. We only need one main meal a day: the rest can be in small snacks taken only when we feel hungry.

You think you cannot make this big change? Then consider the problem of the Japanese Sumo wrestler when he retires. During his fighting years he builds up his enormous weight by grossly overeating. If he continues to eat in the same way after retirement, his life expectancy is very short. So he returns to the normal Japanese style of eating, and the extra weight falls away. Within a year, most are not recognizable as former Sumo wrestlers! If they can do it, so can you!

The right sort of exercise

If you have angina, advice to exercise more probably seems ludicrous. After all, doesn't exercise do precisely what you wish to avoid – bring on the pain? And isn't rest important for your heart? Look what happened to James Fixx!

As I wrote in Chapter 1, James Fixx was actually a success story. He probably gave himself an extra 20 years of worthwhile life before he succumbed to heart disease – and he might well have lived even longer if he had heeded his warning signs and sought medical help.

The fact is that the news about exercise for heart patients is all good. Exercise *is* good for you, even if your heart has been damaged by a previous heart attack. This will surprise many older people, who remember the days when 'heart' patients were advised to rest all the time, and became chair-bound or bedridden on the advice of their doctors. When I was a medical student in the early 1960s, victims of heart attacks were kept in bed for between six and twelve weeks.

The idea was that if you 'rested' the heart until the scar of the attack healed, the scar would be stronger and smaller, and the eventual recovery would be better. From then on, though, the patient was expected to lead a quiet life.

This advice was a hangover from the Victorian age, when it was fashionable to 'take to your bed'. From the mid-1850s right up to the 1960s, people recovering from illnesses and operations were sent to 'convalescent homes' where they rested and lazed around until they were better. It sometimes took a very long time. Charles Darwin and Florence Nightingale spent many years languishing in bed during the daytime, suffering from 'neurasthenia' or 'nervous exhaustion'.

This attitude to rest, and advice against exercise, turned many people into 'cardiac cripples'. They were told they were 'delicate', and must not over-exert themselves. All sorts of activities were forbidden to them, including walking upstairs, running and lovemaking.

None of this advice was based on fact. Some eminent physician had once decreed that this was the way to behave if you were a 'heart' patient, and everyone believed the advice and followed it.

Not today, though. We now know that the more we use an organ, the more effective it becomes, and the heart is no exception even when it is affected by atheroma. It needs to be stimulated to keep strong. If the heart works at resting pace all the time, then it makes it difficult to step up a gear when that is needed.

Today, we aim to keep people with angina as active as their condition allows. You will be asked to walk on a 'treadmill', a moving pavement that can be set at different speeds on the level or on an upward slope, to assess how much you can do, initially, before the heart begins to complain.

While on the treadmill, your heart is monitored by ECG, to pick up changes before the pain starts, and, especially if you have diabetes, to pick up any periods of 'silent' ischaemia (see Chapter 2). You will then be given a programme of exercise to start that will allow you to exercise up to the correct limit, and not beyond. Don't let that scare you. When you add regular exercise to all the other actions you have been taking, such as eating more healthily, stopping smoking and lowering your blood pressure, you will be improving your heart's supply–demand equation all the time. Even people with severe heart failure have been helped by exercise. You will be amazed how quickly you will be able to step up your exercise, and how much better you feel.

7
Taking up – and keeping up – exercise

If you spend a lot of your time sitting down, this chapter is for you. However, even if you feel that you have a lot of exercise, this may not be the right type of exercise, so this chapter is for you too!

Women and exercise

I write a regular column in the *Sunday Mail*, the most widely read Sunday newspaper in Scotland. In August 1995, I wrote about the sad fact that Scottish women, on the whole, appear to be becoming 'couch potatoes'. Over the last 20 years, they have been getting fatter, taking less exercise, and younger women are actually smoking *more* – the reverse of the trend everywhere else, which is that more people are *giving up* smoking.

I pointed out that in the Great Scottish Run, a half-marathon held on 20 August in 1995, that only one-fifth of the 7,200 runners were women, and I challenged them to improve that statistic in 1996.

I expected, and received, a few pointed letters from readers, but the gist of them was disappointing. Most of the women who wrote to me stressed that by the time they had done their own jobs, and added to that the housework and cooking, they were too tired to exercise, far less run half-marathons!

I understand their point and sympathize, but they were in fact shooting the messenger without listening to the message! It is up to women, if they also go out to work, to make sure that their menfolk share the household jobs. That should free them to use their leisure time more effectively, together. If they are full-time housewives, then they can arrange their time to exercise appropriately.

The 'Harvard Step Test'

The most frequent excuse for not doing exercise is that 'after a hard day's work, I just want to crash out on the couch'. That isn't a valid excuse, though. Take half-an-hour or so resting after getting home, sure, but then think about organizing some sort of physical activity.

These days, few jobs are physically demanding, and most employees spend most of their time sitting down. And it is an odd fact that the more time you spend resting, the more you want to rest. It becomes a vicious circle.

So how do you start? First, you can find out how fit your heart is. Try the 'Harvard Step Test' at home. All you need is a bench 20 inches (50 centimetres) high, or a flight of stairs, and a watch with a second hand. You should also know where to find your pulse. It is just above the wrist on the thumb side of the forearm, between the first tendon and the bone. Use your index and middle fingers to time it.

Now step on to the bench or the second step, missing out the first one, and down again, 30 times a minute for 4 minutes. Time yourself with the watch, or use a metronome. You must straighten your knee fully at each step.

If you get too exhausted to carry on, or you feel any chest pain, tightness, discomfort or breathlessness, stop immediately and rest. Note the time you stopped: it makes a difference to your score.

As soon as you have finished, whether you have stopped early or have managed the full 4 minutes, sit down quietly for exactly 1 minute, then time your pulse for 30 seconds. Write down the number of beats. Repeat the 30-second pulse count at 2 minutes, then 3 minutes, after stopping the exercise.

You can then calculate your 'recovery index'. This is the duration of the exercise in seconds multiplied by 100 divided by double the sum of the three pulse counts. This is not as complicated as it sounds!

The following three examples may make the calculation clearer. Mr A, who takes little exercise, stopped after 3 minutes 40 seconds (220 seconds) and had 30-second pulse rates of 76 at 1 minute, 64 at 2 minutes and 60 at 3 minutes. This gives a score of 22,000 (220 seconds x 100) divided by 400 (400 is double his total pulse rates of 76, 64 and 60), which gives the figure of 55. Miss B, who attends an aerobics class twice a week, completed the 4 minutes and had pulse readings of 60 at 1 minute, 52 at 2 minutes and 40 at 3 minutes. Her score (24,000 divided by 320) was 75. Mr C, in his mid-fifties, who runs 5–8 miles three times a week, and runs half-marathons for charity, completed the 4 minutes with 30–second pulse rates of 47 at 1 minute, 39 at 2 minutes and 38 at 3 minutes. His score (24,000 divided by 248) was 97.

Mr A is decidedly unfit, and needs to do better. Miss B could be considered as being of good average fitness. Mr C's score, of well above 90, indicates that he is an athlete in training. If your score is 60 or less, you need to be much fitter. Your fitness is only 'fair' if you score between 61 and 70, 'good' between 71 and 80, and 'very good' between 81 and 90.

Getting fitter

Start off by making the right decision. Don't listen to that voice inside you that says 'I'll get round to it sometime', or 'I've tried to before and couldn't keep it up', or 'I can't make the change just now'. You *can* make the change, even if it is just with a first small step.

There are a few rules for beginning exercise:

1 Start easily and gently, and build up your activity slowly and gradually.
2 Choose an exercise you will enjoy, one that feels right for you.
3 Do exercise that involves your large muscles in your legs, such as in brisk walking, cycling and swimming.
4 Be sensible about starting and stopping. Listen to your body, and don't overdo things.
5 If you have a health problem, such as angina, discuss with your doctor the best type and amount of exercise for you.
6 Do *not* exercise if you are unwell – for example, if you have a throat infection or flu.
7 Do not exercise if you have a muscle strain or injury. Wait until it is pain-free before you start again, and do so slowly.

The best exercise to start with is simply to walk. This is the exercise that benefits our health with the least fuss. Whatever our age and occupation, we can 'take our hearts for a walk'. We don't have to walk far or fast to begin with. The initial aim is to walk for up to 20 minutes three times a week.

You can do it by walking to work or the shops, or walk, rather than drive, to the station. Don't make yourself suffer in bad weather: you won't keep it up, and it may put you off the idea of walking. If you normally catch a bus, get off a stop or two before your own stop, and walk the rest of the way. If you have a dog, take it for a walk yourself, rather than telling the children to do so. Walk at weekends, with the family, to the park, or in the countryside.

Whenever you can, climb stairs rather than use the lift. Walk, rather than drive, to any destination within a mile of your home. Even throw away the remote control of your television set, so that you have to get up to change the programme! *Do* things, rather than watch television, in your spare time. If you do stay at home, try gardening or doing the odd jobs needed around the house.

If you feel you can't keep up your new activities, recognize that it's always easier to start something new than to keep it going. That is why you must choose an activity that you *like*, then start it gently and increase it slowly. Don't despair if you back-slide on a particular exercise. Start again, and keep on starting, because your heart will benefit every time that you do.

Frankly, I'm against the new policy of all-seated football stadia, because I know plenty of men whose only exercise was jumping up and down with excitement or rage at what was happening on the pitch! If you go regularly to the Saturday match, at least walk to the ground, rather than drive or catch the bus.

Once you have started on the exercise programme, you will soon begin to feel better. You will be carrying less weight around, which will be less work for your heart for the same exercise – the demand side of that supply–demand equation is getting better. Your heart and muscles are working more efficiently with the training, and your circulation will be improving. So where do we go from here?

Aerobic fitness

The 'in' word for exercise in the 1990s is aerobics. Aerobic fitness is a measure of how well your heart, lungs and blood vessels get oxygen to your muscles – in other words, your stamina. You become fitter aerobically by using your larger muscles continuously for a relatively long time. You don't do so by stopping and starting a lot, as in gardening, golf or washing your car. You do become fitter if you continue your exercise until you get slightly out of breath, but can still keep up a conversation.

That is what you should aim at – an exercise lasting around 20 minutes that makes you slightly out of breath, three or four times a week. Don't be disheartened if you can't manage it yet, but aim to build up gradually towards that point. Even walking faster than usual for a few minutes is a start towards it, and week by week you will be surprised how much further you can walk before you get to the breathlessness point.

If you are so breathless that you cannot keep up a conversation, or your muscles are getting heavy or sore, then you are working too hard. You will not improve your fitness by exhausting yourself in this way. It is *not* true that exercise needs to hurt your muscles before it does you good. Muscles that are sore are being starved of oxygen, and that is *not* the aim!

Obeying this rule means that you should control your own level of exercise, and not be controlled by some outside influence, like the rhythm of music on a tape, or the need to compete with yourself (by, for example, timing your walking speed or distance).

Don't do too much too quickly. No matter what your exercise, whether it is walking, cycling, running or swimming, don't push yourself to go further each time you do it. If your chosen exercise becomes like hard work, you are more likely to give it up, and the more likely you are to be injured. Your aim is to continue for life, and not for just a few weeks.

Running

If you think you may enjoy running, then by all means try it – but buy the right shoes first. If you intend to run on roads or pavements, you must wear proper road-running shoes with air-cushioned soles. Hard surfaces and the wrong shoes can badly jar ankle, knee and hip joints, to say nothing of the spine.

Running, however, doesn't suit everyone. If you are overweight, then walk or swim instead, until you are nearer a normal shape. Then, if you feel like it, you can start running. Don't start running if you have trouble in the weight-bearing joints – the knees, ankles, hips and back. Swimming and cycling is probably better for you.

If you find the running begins to get boring after a while, change to something else. You will not keep up any exercise for a lifetime if you don't really like it.

Don't become an 'exercise bore'!

Don't take the exercise too seriously, either. 'Exercise bores', who can talk about nothing other than their times and speeds, are hardly popular! In fact, don't buy a stopwatch: competitions and speeds should not be part of your approach. How long you spend on your exercise is probably more important than its intensity. A 4 mile (6 kilometre) walk will get your heart as fit as if you had run the same distance in half the time.

Choose your exercise carefully

Exercise won't kill you, but choose it wisely. Don't opt for explosive exercise, such as weightlifting. The action of lifting weights or straining muscles while holding your breath is harmful, not beneficial. Doctors call it the Valsalva manoeuvre. If you are not a fully trained weightlifter, it can cause a sudden drop in the blood returning from the lower body to the heart. At best it can make you dizzy and faint, at worst it can make you unconscious. If you already have a poor flow of blood through a coronary artery, then the Valsalva manoeuvre can be the final insult, bringing on a heart attack. The same may occur in explosive sports like squash. Golf is more leisurely, and probably better.

If you are thinking of taking up a sport, take a few lessons from a professional first. It will give you an idea of how you will like it, and make it much easier to enjoy. Few 'rabbits' last long in tennis or golf clubs if their skills do not quickly improve.

Warming up for exercise

Whatever the exercise you eventually take up, always warm up first. Warming up raises your body temperature, getting your circulation going, and gently stretches the muscles you will be using. It will help to extend your joint movements, making you less stiff. Even if you are only walking, think of the first five or ten minutes as your warm-up period, easing gently into the walk before striding out and swinging your arms.

A good set of warm-up exercises to do in the 10–15 minutes before your true exercise session is as follows:

1 A very easy run or a walk on the spot for 5 minutes.

2 Then give about 15 seconds to each of the following:

(a) sit in a chair, stretch forward, then stand up several times;

(b) lie on your back, and raise each knee to your chin alternately;

(c) stand with your hands straight out against a wall, and press against it several times;

(d) holding on to the back of a chair, stretch one leg, and then the other straight backwards, keeping the rear foot and heel on the ground, stretching your calf muscles;

(e) lie on your side and bend your upper knee so that the heel comes to the buttock; switch to lie on the other side, and do the same with the other leg;

(f) sit up with one leg straight out and one bent up. Let the bent leg drop sideways to the floor, tucking the foot along the other thigh. Lean forward with arms straight forward out from the shoulder. Do the same with the other leg; this will stretch the groin muscles;

(g) sit up with arms straight in front of you, then turn the trunk until they are at right angles to the legs; then reach down as far as is comfortable;

(h) standing up, raise one arm above your head, then lean over to that side; do the same with the other arm;

(i) stretch both arms as far as you can above your head;

(j) link your arms behind the small of your back with elbows in, and raise your arms in this position.

The do's and don't's of exercise include the following:

DO:

- Choose a sensible programme for yourself, knowing your limitations.

- Warm up for 10 to 15 minutes.

- Ease gently into your exercise, and feel comfortable with it.

- Hold stretches for 15 to 20 seconds.

- Cool down afterwards for 10 to 15 minutes.

DON'T:

- Exercise at a level that is too difficult.
- Stretch cold muscles.
- Force movement or create pain.
- Bounce when stretching.
- Stop suddenly.

You should slow down gradually after any activity, and particularly after running. Ease off near the end, rather than finish with a sprint. Then walk to help your muscles relax gradually. If the exercise has been particularly vigorous, cool down using the same warm-up exercises with which you started.

Don't overdo it!

Don't overdo the exercise. If you have started off at the normal weight for your height, and you find you are losing a pound or two, you are either doing too much or not eating enough to replace the lost energy. Don't replace the heart attack risk with the problems of anorexia nervosa. James Fixx wrote that the best runners looked too thin. They may do, but your objective is not to be one of the best runners. Your aim is to enjoy your exercise while getting your heart as fit as possible. Being a beanpole has disadvantages, and is not necessarily as good for you as being in the normal BMI range – i.e. an average build. Of course, if you start by being overweight, losing the extra pounds through exercise is a bonus, provided that when you reach your ideal weight, you stay at it.

Another 'don't' is to get too obsessional about your weight. I don't recommend regular weighing, as it tends to focus on that one aspect of health, to the exclusion of others. It can cause disappointment, sometimes even despair, if the pounds do not roll off quickly and steadily. That is a mistake, because the exercise will alter your body shape, making you leaner and trimmer, without necessarily causing your weight to change much. Your fat is being replaced by more muscle tissue – and that is more important than losing weight in itself.

So instead of focusing on your weight, follow your progress by looking in a long mirror once in a while. You will know better from your shape and your muscle tone that you are improving, and that will boost your confidence rather than undermine it.

The importance of rest

Daily exercise is all very well, but rest is important too. Some people find that exercise helps them to relax and reduce their stress, because they always 'glow' and feel good after vigorous physical activity. However, they must not exercise vigorously every day.

For muscles, including the heart muscle, to get the best out of exercise, you should take two days of rest from it every week. Plan your week accordingly for two separate 'do little' days between exercises. Professional sportsmen know this – and it is even more important if you have angina.

Rest is important at certain times in your exercise days too. Don't, for example, exercise vigorously for at least two hours after a main meal, or until an hour after a snack. Don't exercise after drinking alcohol (more about this later).

If you are ill, don't try to keep up the exercise schedule, especially if you have a virus infection such as flu or a cold. As you begin to recover, start with a few easy exercises at home – they will help your muscles to recover faster.

Don't stick to just one exercise either. Mix your exercises with walking, swimming, cycling, running, golfing, tennis, badminton, or whatever – whatever you most enjoy. Keep it moderate, and not too competitive, and learn how to relax.

Relaxation techniques

Some people find it easy to relax – they can fall asleep at will when they sit in a chair. Others find it difficult: their minds are racing around some problem or other, and their muscles are tense. If you can spend a few minutes every day in a completely relaxed state, this will complement your exercise schedule, and improve your chances of avoiding the next attack of angina.

The following relaxation technique takes about 10 minutes, and can be done anywhere, even at work. It has helped many patients, and I recommend it:

1 Find a quiet place.

2 Sit in a chair with good back support and with your feet on the floor.
3 Rest your fingers on your stomach and close your eyes.
4 Breathe in and out slowly and gently so that your stomach rises and falls.
5 Take one slow, deep breath.
6 Hold the breath for a slow count of four.
7 Breathe out slowly and steadily, while relaxing all your muscles, and saying to yourself 'relax'.
8 Repeat the sequence as many times as you wish, always slowly, without strain.

It can be difficult to know whether your muscles are fully relaxed or not. One way to learn how to relax them is, paradoxically, to tense them, so that you know how that feels. If you find relaxing difficult, try the following for around 15 minutes a day:

1 Lie down on your back with your arms by your sides on a comfortable floor, and a book under your head so that it is not tilted backwards and your chin is not dipped down towards your chest.
2 Tense up one group of muscles – start with your neck muscles.
3 Notice what the tension in these muscles feels like.
4 Relax the muscles.
5 Notice the different feeling in the muscles now that they are relaxed.
6 Let these feelings and the relaxation increase.
7 Do the same with the rest of your muscle groups, throughout the whole body, one at a time. Plan your own way around your body – I start with the right arm, then the left, the neck, scalp, face, shoulders, back, chest, stomach, right leg and left leg.

If you would like to learn more formal ways to relax, try yoga or Tai Chi, the slow exercises favoured by the Chinese. A 1995 study in Britain comparing the benefits of various forms of relaxation found Tai Chi the most effective in lowering blood pressure and heart rate.

The benefits for your heart

Apart from feeling better and looking better, what does regular exercise do for the heart?

It has been shown, and this is about the one point on which all the experts on heart disease do agree, that it reduces the risk of, or postpones the onset of, a whole series of diseases, including arthritis, rheumatism, disc trouble, diabetes, high blood pressure, coronary disease, stroke, and even depression and anxiety. And if you are overweight, it is the best way to lose the flab.

If you exercise regularly you are less likely to smoke and overeat (exercise does *not* make you hungry, or eat more). Your blood pressure falls and your heart beats more slowly and more efficiently at rest. When you exercise, the heart rate rises slower, to a lower peak, and returns to normal faster if you are a regular exerciser than if you are a 'couch potato'. That means the supply–demand equation so often mentioned in this book is tilted to your benefit.

Exercising regularly also postpones the onset of old age. You can recognize old people who have exercised regularly by their straighter backs, their better neck movements, their more mobile joints and more bulky muscles. They are fitter mentally, too, being less depressed and less isolated from others.

Exercise is particularly important for women. It helps to drive calcium into their bones, so warding off the excesses of osteoporosis, the disease that causes 60,000 older women in Britain every year to have fractured hips. For these women, calcium loss from bones can be a serious problem after the menopause. Physically active women start off their menopause with a bigger 'bank' of calcium in their thigh and hip bones, so that any later loss of calcium, hopefully, is never so severe that these bones will break.

It is never too late to start exercising, for men or women. For more than 20 years now, heart attack survivors have been encouraged to exercise as soon as they have recovered from the experience. There have been some astonishing successes. Dr Terence Kavanagh, who ran a Cardiac Rehabilitation Centre in Toronto, encouraged his patients to start carefully, building up to a light jog for an hour at a time.

Marathons and half-marathons

Some of Dr Kavanagh's patients suggested that they try a marathon – marathons being popular at the time. He was doubtful at first, but then encouraged them. After careful training, all seven of his first group of patients finished the 26-mile (41-kilometre) journey with no ill effects. They then presented him with a trophy inscribed 'Super-coach, the World's Sickest Track Club'!

Of course, marathons are for a very select group of people, and no one with angina should attempt one unless he or she has first had the full treatment to minimize any possible harmful effect. And the enthusiasm for the general public to enter marathons has died away in the 1990s – rightly so, because too many untrained amateurs were being put at serious health risk.

However, half-marathons are still popular. I ran in the Great Scottish Run in August 1995, and thought I had put up a creditable performance, finishing in about 1 hour 55 minutes on an amazingly hot day for Scotland. The temperature was in the nineties (Fahrenheit) (thirties Centigrade) for the last hour of the race, so I found the last mile and a half wearing, to say the least. I was amazed to find that one of my patients had finished 20 minutes before me, feeling fit and comfortable. A year before he had had a triple bypass operation for severe angina!

Of course, he could never have achieved his run without the new coronary circulation. Nor could he have done it without the determination to get well again. He used exercise to do it. I do not suggest that half-marathon running is the choice for more than a very few people, but there is always some exercise that you can do to improve things – and it is much better than sitting around worrying about the future! And that is often the alternative.

Prove to yourself the benefits of exercise

You can prove to yourself the benefits of exercise. Do the 'Harvard Step Test' described at the beginning of this chapter now, then try the exercise of your choice for a week, then do the Step Test again. You will be surprised how much your score will have improved in that short time. It will be easier to continue for the full 4 minutes, and your pulse rates will be much slower. Keep going, and aim eventually to maintain yourself in the mid-70 region. You do not have to be an Olympic athlete to be fit and well.

8
Smoking

If you are a non-smoker, you can skip this chapter, unless you wish to be armed with all the material you need to stop other people from lighting up. If you are a smoker, but have been convinced to stop by what I have already written, then read on. You may be helped to stop permanently by what you read. If you still have doubts about whether you can stop, read this chapter again and again. It could well save your life.

Smoking and angina

If you don't want to stop, and you have angina, then you may as well give this book away and put your affairs in order. If you continue to smoke, your chances of surviving for any length of time are slim. No matter what else you do to protect your heart, it is being overwhelmed by your suicidal habit of smoking.

If you could invent something that in every way was guaranteed to give you angina and a heart attack, then smoking would be it. It reduces the oxygen levels in your blood, it narrows further your already narrowed coronary arteries, it poisons your heart muscle with carbon monoxide and your brain with nicotine, it makes your blood very much more likely to clot, and it directly damages your most delicate blood vessels.

Yet I have known many patients continue to smoke after a coronary bypass or a heart attack. I'm sure that they do not wish to kill themselves, but that is exactly what they are doing. It is so unfair to their families, and even to non-smokers who are waiting for their own bypass operations, and who will benefit far more from the skill and devotion of their surgeons.

Smoking gives people a sallow unhealthy look, and wrinkles. By the time they are 40, women smokers look ten years older than their non-smoking counterparts. By the time they are 60, many of them are already dead. Cancer of the lung and heart attacks, both of them directly due to smoking, cause far more early deaths in women than anything else.

Most smokers lit their first cigarette as teenagers, when they were far too immature to think about the long-term risk. If you are a non-smoker at 20, it is odds on that you will remain so for the rest of your life. By this time, most people have learned sense!

If you have angina and still smoke, it is not too late to learn sense. To a doctor like myself, who has had to comfort so many families in which smoking has directly led to the deaths of men and women in their forties and fifties, it is frankly incredible that anyone should ever wish to light up a single cigarette. For a smoker who mulls over the facts about his or her habit, continuing to smoke means that cigarettes mean more than life itself – yet 40 per cent of the population continue to smoke them.

So the rest of this chapter aims to dissuade you from the use of tobacco for the rest of your life. Consider the following facts:

- Heart attacks are the inevitable end of the road for an angina sufferer who continues to smoke.

- Smoking causes more deaths from heart attacks than it does deaths from any other cause, including chronic bronchitis and lung cancer.

- People who smoke cigarettes have two or three times the risk of a fatal heart attack than non-smokers. The more they smoke, the greater the risk.

- Men under 45 who smoke 25 or more cigarettes a day have 10 to 15 times the chance of dying from a heart attack than non-smokers.

- In developed countries such as Britain, one-third of men die before they reach 65, mainly from smoking-related diseases.

- One-third of all married women are widows before they can enjoy retirement with their husbands, mainly because their husbands smoked.

- About 40 per cent of all heavy smokers die before they reach 65. Of the 60 per cent of smokers still alive at that age, many are disabled by bronchitis, angina, heart failure or because they have had a leg amputated.

- Of all smokers, only 10 per cent reach 75 years of age. Most non-smokers reach age 75 in good health.

- Smoking takes a terrible toll in ways other than heart attacks. In Britain, 40 per cent of all cancer deaths in men are due to lung cancer. It is very rare in non-smokers. Of 441 British male doctors who died of lung cancer, only seven had never smoked. Only one non-smoker in 60 develops lung cancer (even that case is probably caused by passive smoking): the figure for heavy smokers is one in six!

- Women smokers, too, get lung cancer. It has recently overtaken breast cancer in Britain as the cancer causing most deaths in women. And young women are now more likely to be smokers than young men. What a catastrophe that conjures up for the next generation!

- Other cancers more common in smokers than in non-smokers include tumours of the tongue, throat, larynx, pancreas, kidney, bladder and cervix. About one-third of all cancers are caused directly by smoking.

- Don't think that because you have angina, you won't get one of these other smoking-related diseases as well. Many smokers have multiple diseases, all caused by their love for cigarettes.

So take stock now if you have angina and you still smoke. You can't use the false hope of so many people when they face the future – 'It may not happen to me' – because it *has* happened to you! You have already been damaged by your habit, and you can be damaged far more if you continue. Nor should you use the excuses heard by every doctor. They are listed here, with their honest answers:

- *My father/grandfather/uncle smoked 20 a day and lived until he was 75.*

Everyone knows someone like that. But they forget all the others they knew who died long before their time. The chances are, if you continue to smoke, that you will be one of them, and not one of the very few survivors.

- *People who don't smoke also have angina.*

True, there are other causes of heart attacks, but 70 per cent of all people under 65 years old admitted to coronary care units with heart attacks are smokers, as are 91 per cent of patients considered for bypass surgery.

• *Moderation in all things is acceptable: I only smoke moderately.*

That is rubbish. Do people accept moderation in lead poisoning, dangerous driving, radiation or exposure to asbestos (which causes many fewer deaths than smoking)? Of course not. Younger men who are 'moderate' smokers have a much higher risk of heart attack than non-smokers of the same age. There is no lower safe limit to smoking.

• *I can cut down rather than stop.*

You may be able to, but it won't do much good. Smokers who cut down usually take more inhalations from each cigarette, leaving a smaller butt, and end up with the same amount of carbon monoxide and nicotine in the bloodstream. The only answer is to stop.

• *I am just as likely to be run over in the road as to die from smoking.*

This is ridiculous. In Britain, about 12 people die on the roads each day. This compares with 100 a day from lung cancer, 100 from chronic bronchitis and 100 from heart attacks. Almost all of these deaths are directly due to smoking. Of every 1,000 young men who smoke, on average one will be murdered, six will die on the roads, and 250 will die before their time from smoking.

• *I have to die of something.*

In my experience this is always said by someone in good health, and not by someone who has developed angina or has had a heart attack. It is definitely *never* said by someone who has started to cough up blood!

• *I don't want to be old anyway.*

We define 'old' differently as we grow older! Most of us would like to live a long time, but none of us wants to be old and infirm. If we take care of ourselves on the way to being old, we have at least laid the groundwork for a good chance of enjoying our old age. Smoking destroys that chance for the vast majority.

• *I'd rather die of a heart attack than from anything else.*

Most of us would like to die in a 'clean' way. But many heart attack victims leave grieving partners in their early fifties to face 20 or 30 years of loneliness. Is that what you would wish?

- *Stress, not smoking, is the main cause of angina and heart attacks.*

Who has the most stress? The top executive or the single parent on a low income struggling to make ends meet? Stress is not only difficult to measure, it is very difficult to relate to angina in any meaningful way. In any case, the stress is there to be coped with somehow: smoking is an extra burden on your heart that can never help.

- *I'll stop if I have a heart attack.*

That would be fine if first heart attacks were not fatal within four hours in 40 per cent of people! It is too late to think of stopping smoking then!

- *I'll put on weight if I stop smoking.*

You probably will, because your appetite will return and you will be able to taste food again. So take the opportunity to make the change in your eating habits described earlier. If you do put on weight, it will only be temporary. In any case, the health risks of putting on a few pounds are far lower than those of continuing to smoke.

- *I enjoy smoking, and don't want to give it up.*

Is that really true, or is it just an excuse to cover up the fact that you can't stop? What is your real pleasure in smoking? Be honest with yourself.

- *Cigarettes settle my nerves. If I didn't smoke, I would have to take Valium.*

Smoking is certainly a prop, like a baby's dummy. The packet, the lighter, the fondling of the cigarette, holding it in the mouth, the need to do something with the hands, are all part of the ritual that seems to be needed by the smoker. But it solves nothing. It does not remove the cause of any stress, and can only make things worse in the long run because of its bad effect on health. There are other, much healthier, ways of dealing with your nervousness.

As you continue to smoke, the ritual of the habit takes up more of your time, making you less efficient, less energetic, and causing you to lose your enjoyment of other pleasures, like food. Non-smoking friends feel freer nowadays to object to your habit, and you are likely to have to leave your workplace to indulge in it outside. In Finland, you would have to go at least 15 metres away from your office door! All these little things tend to increase your anxiety, so that with each cigarette you are reminded of the damage you may be doing. Surely it would be better to stop altogether – you would then be in much less stressful circumstances. Interestingly, the anxiety-prone smoker who worries about it has a better than average chance of giving up.

- *I'll change to a pipe or cigars – they are safer.*

Not for you, they aren't. Lifelong pipe and cigar smokers are at very little increased risk of a heart attack, but they still have five times the lung cancer rate and ten times more chronic bronchitis than non-smokers. Cigarette smokers who switch to pipes or cigars, unfortunately, continue to be at high risk of a heart attack, probably because they still inhale.

- *I've been smoking for years, so it is too late to stop.*

No, it is not, at whatever age you stop, no matter how long you have been smoking. The risk of a sudden death from a heart attack drops steeply if you stop smoking, becoming close to the non-smoker's risk in two to three years. If you carry on smoking after a heart attack, make sure that your life insurance is in order. Stopping smoking also reduces your risk of lung cancer, but the fall in risk is slower, reducing by 80 per cent over 15 years.

- *I wish I could stop. I have tried everything, but nothing has worked.*

Stopping smoking is easy, if you *really* want to do it. But you need to put effort into it yourself, and not expect anyone else to do it for you. This means you must be motivated to stop. If the last few pages have not motivated you, then nothing will!

Reasons for stopping smoking

Reasons for stopping smoking vary from generation to generation. Those teenagers who smoke heed health warnings only rarely – they think the possibility of death is too far away to bother about, and the danger may even attract them. However, they will often listen if a potential partner says that smoking is smelly and dirty, and immature. They will sometimes also listen to the environmental argument, such as that big multinational companies are exploiting Third World poverty to their massive benefit. Pakistan, Zimbabwe and Brazil put hundreds of thousands of acres of fertile land, which could be used for food, under tobacco, to serve the appetite of the developed world for tobacco. That profit does not reach the average person in these tobacco-producing countries.

Even worse, the tobacco companies are vigorously promoting their deathly products to the poorer countries, adding lung and heart diseases to their already huge health problems. What right-minded person can collude in that process? Ask any teenager!

The appearance of a smoker can be another powerful motive to stop. Smoking induces wrinkles and a grey, pasty complexion. Women who smoke could save themselves the horrendous costs of beauty creams and of cigarettes, *and* look far better by stopping smoking.

For older men and women, and particularly people with angina, the main motivation to stop must be health. Remember the statistics given a few pages ago. They are horrific for the smoker with angina. A third of all men do not live to collect their pensions, mainly because of their smoking. There are few 'merry widows' outside of opera – that fact alone should be enough to make people stop. But how to do it?

How to stop smoking

Five years ago, I was advising people that they had a choice in stopping: they could stop suddenly or gradually. Now I'm convinced that the first is the only way, and I advise the 'General de Gaulle' method.

General de Gaulle announced to the whole French nation, on television, that he had stopped smoking. After that, he could hardly light up in case a member of the press caught him and exposed him as a fraud or backslider! Most people could do something similar, in front of friends. Today's anti-smoking climate will ensure their sympathy and support, rather than sneers or sniggers.

I advise people to take all the cigarettes they possess, in pockets, handbags, at home or anywhere else, to scrunch them up, and throw them in the bin or on the fire. They should then resolve never to buy another cigarette, and always say 'no' immediately, without even thinking about it, to anyone who offers them one. If they do not wish to argue with smoking friends, a non-smoking sticker in the car and on the front window of the home can help.

People contemplating suddenly stopping smoking often fear withdrawal symptoms. These symptoms *can* include agitation, irritability, sleeplessness and nervousness – but such things may be completely absent. I have found that people who have to give up for serious medical reasons, such as angina, hardly ever have withdrawal symptoms. If you have decided to stop because of your angina, it is long odds on that you will have no bother with withdrawal. You may still have a desire to smoke, but that will subside in a week or two, as your new feeling of well-being, caused by the elimination from the bloodstream of carbon monoxide, nicotine and tar-linked chemicals takes over.

If you must do something else to take your mind off cigarettes, then chew low-calorie gum or, better still, pieces of carrot or celery. Get a friend to support you in the effort.

If you find that you cannot stop first time, don't despair. Try again. Many people find that they have to stop several times before they can do it permanently. You can try acupuncture or hypnosis if you wish, but they do not have any magical properties. They only support your own determination, and cannot overrule weak willpower. If you have angina, you should *not* use nicotine chewing gum or patches. They work by supplying nicotine to your bloodstream, on the principle that it will stop any craving for tobacco. However, that nicotine can still narrow your arteries, and may even promote a heart attack if you 'backslide' and start smoking again. The combination of nicotine from the cigarettes and from the gum or patches may be too much for your heart.

Understand that stopping smoking is not an and in itself. Smoking has been part of your life, probably for many years. It was almost a 'friend' to you. You must replace it with a new positive approach to life, one that takes in your new eating and exercise habits. They will take your mind off the cigarette routine. Eat more fruit, for example. Your rediscovered taste buds will really enjoy it. Try a new hobby, and meet new friends. Avoid places that you know will be smoky, and be on your guard at all times. Resolve never to buy or accept another cigarette. Never risk 'just one', even when you have had alcohol and your resistance is low. Just one cigarette can lead to another, and you will soon be back where you started, in a matter of a few weeks.

If you have angina, you owe making the effort to stop smoking to your heart and your future, and to the future of your partner and your family. You are not alone. Several million Britons have given up the habit in the last ten years. Only one in three British adults now smokes. Now that you have stopped (I assume that having read this far you must have made that decision), you have simply joined the sensible majority.

Action on Smoking and Health (ASH)

As a new non-smoker, you will discover that there are many public places where you cannot avoid breathing in other people's smoke. This will annoy you (possibly more than you ever imagined when you smoked). You can do something about it by contacting ASH (the address is on page 111). ASH has been fighting for years for the rights of non-smokers to breathe in smoke-free air.

It is succeeding. Many offices now ban smoking in the building. I mentioned earlier that I write a weekly column for the *Sunday Mail*; its Glasgow headquarters houses dozens of journalists in an open-plan system. The building has been smoke-free for some years now – and the people working there have enjoyed much better health and working conditions since the ban started.

In October 1993, ASH launched its 'Breathing Space' campaign to create a more smoke-free atmosphere in four areas: at work; in restaurants, cafés and pubs; in public places such as banks and post offices; and in schools. The campaign is strongly supported by many health-related organizations, and is part of the Europe Against Cancer initiative, also launched in 1993.

ASH asked people all over Britain where their own smoke-free areas are, and is creating a detailed library of where people can go to avoid other people's smoke. The process is more advanced in Scandinavia and North America than in Britain, but it is still useful here, and we should soon catch up. Contact ASH if you wish to know more, or even if you wish to take part in the survey.

I am ending this chapter with a list of the practical benefits of stopping smoking, according to the time since you stopped. It should support your decision, and help to maintain you as a smoke-free zone!

- *Within 20 minutes of stopping*

Your blood pressure decreases to the normal range.

Your pulse slows down to a normal rate.

The temperature of our fingers and toes rises to normal.

- *After eight hours*

Carbon monoxide levels in the blood return to normal.

Blood oxygen levels return to normal.

- *After one day*

The chances of your having a heart attack have diminished.

- *After two days*

Your senses of smell and taste are heightened.

Your coronary vessels are much wider.

Your blood is much less likely to clot.

- *After three days*

Your airways (the bronchi) are opened up.

You are breathing easier.

Your heart is much more efficient and less strained.

- *After two weeks to three months*

Walking is easier.

You can exercise for much longer.

Your circulation in your feet and fingers is much improved.

- *After nine months*

Your lungs are free of tars.

You no longer have a morning cough.

- *After five years*

Your annual lung cancer death risk has dropped from 137 to 72 per 100,000.

- *After ten years*

Your annual risk of death from lung cancer has dropped to 12 per 100,000.

You are also at much less risk of cancer of the mouth, throat, oesophagus, bladder, kidney and pancreas.

So enjoy the fact that you are now a non-smoker. You have probably saved your life by making the decision.

9

Alcohol

Is alcohol linked to angina?

Now you are a non-smoker, should you be a non-drinker too? Here the evidence is not so clear. Many studies have tried to relate alcohol consumption to heart disease, and the results have often been surprising. So surprising, in fact, that the message has got around that regular drinking of moderate amounts of alcohol might actually be good for the heart – and that total abstention can raise your risk of angina and heart attack.

Sadly, I have to disabuse the reader of that opinion. Although the evidence does suggest that heart attack deaths are commoner in teetotallers than in drinkers, the difference, if it truly exists, is very small, and is more than made up for by deaths from other causes that *are* directly caused by alcohol.

In theory, alcohol should help the heart. Alcohol tends to open up arteries – hence the drinker's rosy cheeks (and nose!) – so that some doctors have argued that a little alcohol might benefit patients with coronary problems.

However, much depends on how we define 'a little', and on whether the patient can stick to the advice. 'A little' can very easily become 'a lot'!

The King's College Hospital guidelines on alcohol

Probably the team to have done more than any other to investigate the effects and ill-effects of different amounts of alcohol is that led by Professor Roger Williams, who was based at the Liver Unit at London's King's College Hospital for more than twenty years until he retired in 1995. This team's study of the drinking habits of thousands of people have led to guidelines that have been accepted all over the world.

Doctors have accepted for many years that the main organs

attacked by alcohol are the liver and the brain. Heavy drinking leads to cirrhosis and cancer of the Liver, and can lead to a 'toxic encephalopathy' in which the brain degenerates, leading to dementia and psychosis. It is also associated with cancers of the stomach and pancreas. However, until recently, it has not been particularly linked with heart disease.

How much is 'too much' alcohol? The King's College team have defined standard units of alcohol. One unit is equivalent to a half-pint (500 ml) of beer or lager, one glass of wine, one measure of fortified wines such as sherry or martini, and a single measure of spirit, such as whisky or gin (a 'half' measure in Scotland).

Men, it is advised, can cope with up to 20 standard drinks a week, and women up to 12. The difference is not just to do with their relative sizes, but to the fact that women's livers have less capacity than men's to deal with alcohol. This means that the regular male drinker should take no more than three drinks per day, and the female drinker no more than two drinks per day. Even this may be too much if the drinking occurs every day. Professor Williams's team recommend that we give our bodies a rest from alcohol on at least three days a week.

This advice was originally given to help people avoid liver and brain damage, but it is now seen as important for the heart too. Alcohol in itself is not thought to cause angina or heart attacks, in that it does not cause arteries to narrow or accelerate the process of atheroma, or make the blood more viscous. By opening up blood vessels, it even gained a reputation for being helpful to the heart. Unfortunately, that reputation was wrong.

Alcohol and blood pressure

Dr Gareth Beevers, of Dudley Road Hospital, Birmingham, is highly respected internationally for his work on high blood pressure. His review of thousands of people with high blood pressure showed a very strong link between alcohol consumption and high blood pressure. The more people drank, the higher were their blood pressures.

This finding flew in the face of the accepted wisdom on alcohol. After all, a substance that opened up blood vessels would be expected to lower pressure, not raise it. Dr Beevers showed that the pressure-raising effect was due to a direct action of alcohol on the heart muscle itself, even when it was taken in moderate amounts. Many moderate drinkers had enlarged hearts, high blood pressure and a poor heart reserve in times of illness.

Dr Beevers's conclusion was that if you have angina, alcohol will always make that worse rather than better. It is safer for people with angina, he concluded, to be teetotal than to drink even a moderate amount.

So how much alcohol can a person drink without harming health? The King's College rules still apply to men and women who have no sign of liver, brain or heart disease. If you have angina, and especially if you have high blood pressure too, then the 20 a week total for men and the 12 a week total for women may be too much. Each case is different. My advice, if you have angina, is to discuss your drinking habits fully and honestly with your cardiologist, who will guide you on what is best for you.

Research on alcohol and angina and heart disease

That guidance may be based not just on the work of Professor Williams and Dr Beevers, but also on the most recent results of the many studies of the possible links between alcohol and heart disease. Unfortunately, the results are far from clear, and many different conclusions have been drawn from them.

Probably the most reliable conclusions were drawn by Professor A.G. Shaper, of the British Regional Heart Study mentioned in the Introduction, in 1994. This showed that moderate drinkers (16–42 units a week) suffered 34 per cent fewer deaths from heart attack, and 13 per cent fewer deaths from other circulation disorders (mainly stroke) than non-drinkers.

This would seem to be encouraging for drinkers – but Professor Shaper stressed that it was not. First, the actual over-all numbers of such deaths were so small that the differences could not be considered as reliable or 'statistically significant'. Worse, there was no reduction in over-all death rate among the moderate drinkers, so that they were more likely to die from other diseases at the same time.

Professor Shaper showed that the extra heart deaths among the teetotallers included several in people who had been diagnosed as having heart disease when they entered the study. They may well have been drinkers who had turned teetotal because they were already feeling ill, and this could account for the difference in death rates. He concluded that if moderate drinking does protect against heart attacks, the effect is relatively small, and is not accompanied by a reduction in deaths from all types of circulation disorders, or by a reduction in deaths over all.

He compared his results with those of studies in other countries. In Trinidad, the lowest mortality for all causes was in men labelled as 'abstemious', who did not usually drink, and had no history of drinking problems. In the large 'Kaiser Permanente' study in the United States, which used lifelong abstainers as a comparison, none of the drinking groups – ranging from occasional, through mild, moderate and heavy – showed any benefit from their alcohol consumption, and those drinking more than six units a day were decidedly worse off.

In a study carried out by the American Cancer Society, in the data on deaths from all causes, only occasional drinkers and those taking one or two drinks a day had a signficantly lower risk than non-drinkers. Here, too, the figures may be distorted by some people who gave up drinking because they were already unwell before they entered the study. Above the lowest alcohol intake level, death rates rose progressively with each step up in alcohol consumption.

In this same study, at the level of alcohol intake associated with the lowest risk of coronary heart disease death (four drinks per day), there was an increased risk for all-cause deaths, particularly from accidents and violence, cancer and stroke, which more than out-weighed the apparent savings in 'heart' deaths. This bleak statistic does not take into account the increased rates of illness that may stem from consuming much lower amounts of alcohol than four drinks a day.

Conclusions about alcohol and angina

So what should we conclude about alcohol and angina? Can angina sufferers have the occasional drink? My feeling is that they can, but it has to be under strict control, and probably less than the King's College guidelines for both men and women. I would restrict drinking to the odd glass of wine with meals, and I still recommend abstention for three days a week. If you also have high blood pressure, then I would go further and advise only the very occasional drink as a 'treat'.

A final word about alcohol. Probably the busiest times of the year for family doctors are the days after a national holiday such as Christmas Day in England, or New Year's Eve (Hogmanay) in Scotland. It may be the same after Thanksgiving in the United States. Special occasions for a family, such as a birthday, anniversary, wedding or reunion, provide the same circumstances. At times like these, people over-eat, usually a meal full of fat, and over-drink. Inhibitions are lost, everyone is very happy, and they go to bed full of food and drink.

During the night, all the conditions for shutting down the blood flow through a coronary artery are fulfilled. The extra fat in the bloodstream makes the blood more viscous, and the flow more sluggish. The blood is more likely to clot. The alcohol that you have drunk ensures that the blood pressure remains just a little higher than usual, and the strain on the plaque sitting in your coronary artery is a little greater. The result, in the small morning hours, may well be a heart attack.

I hate to be a killjoy, but if you have taken the trouble to change your lifestyle to protect your heart, it is a pity to throw all the advantages away just because of one night of over-indulgence. You can enjoy a party much better sober than you can even a little drunk – and think of how much better you will feel in the morning.

10

High blood pressure

High blood pressure (hypertension), like cholesterol, smoking and alcohol, deserves a chapter of its own in any book of angina. Hypertension causes complications for the heart in two ways: it directly increases the work done by the heart, so that the demand for oxygen is increased, and it accelerates the process of atheroma, so that the coronary vessels in someone with hypertension are even more affected by atheroma, and therefore narrower, than in someone with normal blood pressure.

Hypertension is linked with higher than normal risks of stroke, heart attack and kidney disease, and it is vital that it should be controlled in anyone with angina. Professor Giuseppe Mancia of the University of Milan, one of the world's leading experts in the study of hypertension, recently spelled out to me the risks of the combination of hypertension and angina.

The combination of hypertension and angina

A raised systolic blood pressure increases the risk of developing heart failure by fivefold, and a raised diastolic pressure raises the stroke risk by seven or eight times and the heart attack risk by three times. Trials have shown that reducing the blood pressure reduces the risk accordingly. Even if the blood pressure is only moderately raised, reducing it to normal levels will reduce the risk of a heart attack or stroke.

The treatment works regardless of age. The European Working Party on Hypertension, of which Professor Mancia was a member, followed 1,000 elderly people with hypertension for seven years who were either taking active blood pressure-reducing drugs or placebo. This is not as unethical as it sounds, for at the time the trial was started, many doctors believed that reducing blood pressure in the elderly might cause more illness than leaving it alone. It was feared that the lower blood pressure might lower the blood flow to the brain and cause thrombosis or memory problems.

The fear proved to be unnecessary. The persons whose blood pressures were lowered had 35 per cent fewer strokes, heart attacks and deaths than those given placebo.

Other trials have since confirmed this result. When an analysis of all the available controlled (i.e. scientifically acceptable) trials was made, treating hypertension led to a halving of deaths from strokes and heart attacks.

From all the results, Professor Mancia calculated how many lives would be saved if all people with hypertension were actively treated to bring their blood pressure down into the normal range. Even using the lowest calculations of benefit, this action would save more than 5,000 lives annually in a country such as Italy, with a population of 55 million people.

Of course, Professor Mancia performed his calculation for his own countrymen, but exactly the same figures apply to the United Kingdom, with a similar population, and very similar figures for hypertension. The true figure of lives saved, Professor Mancia concedes, is probably much greater than 5,000 for the trials may have underestimated the benefit, because some people in the trials were not truly hypertensive, and many people who were supposed to be taking placebo also took antihypertensive drugs! When they found their blood pressures were rising, they switched to active treatment.

One trial in particular is important for angina sufferers. The SHEP (Systolic Hypertension in the Elderly) study showed not only that there was 32 per cent less disease of the heart and circulation in those whose blood pressures were treated with blood pressure-lowering drugs, but that they had fewer heart attacks and had less need for coronary bypass grafts and angioplasty operations. The message is that if you have angina and hypertension, lowering your blood pressure into the normal range and keeping it there is the most important and effective way to stay fit and alive – and, as a bonus, it may enable you to avoid surgery.

If you have diabetes as well

If you have diabetes as well as angina, then keeping the blood pressure under excellent control is even more important. Diabetes and hypertension go hand in hand: more people with diabetes than without it have hypertension. In people with both diseases, very many have angina, and they are at much higher risk of a heart attack than the rest of us. Now we know that treatment to lower their blood pressures is very much more effective at reducing their risks of heart attack and kidney failure than even the most rigorous control of their diabetes itself.

The target

One of the first large studies of the results of blood-pressure lowering, the United Kingdom Medical Research Council Trial, concluded that in high-risk subjects (defined as those with mildly raised diastolic and a high systolic blood pressure, male, smokers and people with a high blood cholesterol) treating the blood pressure would prevent one stroke per four patients over five years. In a low-risk person, with only a mildly raised diastolic pressure and no other risk factors, the saving would be one stroke per 242 patients in the same time period.

That trial used a combination of antihypertensive drugs that is now outdated, and has been superseded by newer drugs, so that treatment for hypertension is even more effective now, and with better chances of saving lives.

How far do you need to bring your blood pressure down? Analysis of 14 major trials of blood pressure treatment showed that reducing the blood pressure by 5–6 mm Hg led to a 14 per cent reduction in heart attacks. This is true whether the initial blood pressure is extremely high or just moderately raised.

This finding was surprising to the researchers, who expected the benefit to be less in patients with less severe hypertension. It has meant that the target figures for a satisfactory blood pressure have been changed. The old target was a diastolic pressure of 90 mm Hg. Then it became 85 mm Hg. Now it is 80 mm Hg or less, and the savings in illness and deaths continue to increase. It appears, for diastolic pressure, that the lower it is, the better.

We can lower our blood pressures to some extent by changing to the healthier lifestyle of good eating and exercise described earlier, but this is not enough for many people with angina and hypertension. These people also need blood pressure-lowering (antihypertensive) drugs. Such drugs will be described in Chapter 12, but if you wish to know more about the subject, you may like to read my book entitled *Living with High Blood Pressure* (1995, Sheldon Press).

11

Managing angina –
entering the heart unit

Once your doctor has made the tentative diagnosis of angina, you will
be asked to undergo tests to confirm it, and to assess the severity of
your problem. Although lifestyle changes as described in the last few
chapters are vital to your eventual well-being, you will almost
certainly need help from medicines and, perhaps, surgery. How your
family doctor and cardiologist come to their decisions on the
management of your angina are explained in this chapter.

First, it is important to accept that your symptoms may bear no
relationship to the severity of your coronary disease. A person with
only minor symptoms – the occasional tightness across the chest on
strenuous exertion – may have very extensive and multiple stenoses
(narrowing) in all three coronary arteries. That person, male or
female, is sitting on a time bomb, and needs urgent help.

Seeing your doctor

So if you suspect you have angina, you *must* seek your doctor's help.
It is the task of your family doctor to try to sort out the cause of your
chest pain or discomfort, and if there is any possibility that it could be
angina, he or she will send you to the local hospital's heart unit (also
called cardiology unit) for further investigation. While you are
waiting for your hospital appointment to come through, you will
probably be given drugs such as a 'nitrate' to relieve any attack in the
meantime, and told to take half an aspirin a day as a preventive
treatment. The reasons for this double treatment will be explained
later.

Your family doctor's judgement will be based on the history you
give of your symptoms, on a physical examination, on simple blood
tests (e.g. to rule out anaemia) and on an electrocardiogram (ECG).
Some family doctors also have access to chest X-ray facilities, so that
the outline of the heart can be examined. You will then be sent to the
cardiology unit with a letter explaining your doctor's findings.

The cardiology unit

The aim of a modern cardiology unit is to find the cause of your symptoms. Most of the time, in angina, this will be atheroma, affecting one, two or all three of your coronary arteries. The tests to be performed in the clinic should identify the problem in sharp detail, so that any corrective treatment is planned for your own individual needs.

You will be asked to undergo exercise testing, special ECG tests and X-ray investigations, including perhaps a radio-isotope heart scan, an echocardiography, and finally a coronary angiogram.

The thought of all those tests, especially after you have been told you may have a 'dicky' heart, is daunting and frightening. Please do not let it worry you. In modern cardiology units, everything is done to make sure you are relaxed and calm. The staff are highly specialized, having concentrated on heart investigations for years, and know very well what entering such a unit means for their patients.

I have visited many such units in Britain and Europe, all of them staffed by cheerful, kind and dedicated nurses and doctors, who can make even the most apprehensive patient feel relaxed. The atmosphere is never sombre – there is no 'gloom and doom'. The feeling is more of a professionalism dedicated to helping people back to a normal life, with much to look forward to. They have every reason to be cheerful, because they succeed in their aims with the vast majority of their patients.

The first investigations aim to find the underlying cause of the symptoms. They will rule out such problems as heart valve disease (one clue being a heart murmur heard through the stethoscope), high blood pressure, an overactive thyroid or anaemia. If patients are found to have one of these problems, they will be given treatment and their angina should recede. Sometimes the heart clinic finds evidence of spasm (a form of cramp) in the oesophagus, and will pass you on to the appropriate expert for treatment.

Most of the rest of the patients seen with angina in the cardiology unit have atheroma affecting the coronary arteries. The next aim is to find out how serious this is, and to estimate the risks of a full blown heart attack in the near future. That means getting as many details as possible of how the heart is performing at the time of an angina attack. The two ways of doing this, initially, are to use a treadmill test or a Holter monitor.

The treadmill and the Holter monitor

The treadmill is a moving walkway, the speed and incline of which can be altered. The faster it moves and the steeper the incline, the more work it forces your heart to do. While you walk on the treadmill, your heart is monitored by ECG, which will show when the demand for oxygen by the heart is beginning to outstrip the supply through the coronary arteries. This is usually well before you feel any pain.

The ECG can show how much of the heart is affected, and which part of the heart. This helps to pinpoint which coronary artery is affected, and roughly where. It is a start on the road to defining what exactly your problem is, but it is too inaccurate to use as the sole basis of treatment.

As a rough rule of thumb, if angina or ischaemic changes on the ECG start within two minutes of beginning the treadmill exercise, there is enough coronary disease for serious note to be taken. If you can go ten minutes without pain, and there is no 'silent' ischaemia on the ECG, there is little to worry about. However, many people fall in between these limits!

The Holter monitor is a portable computerized ECG machine that can be strapped to your chest for 24 or 48 hours. You wear it as you perform your everyday tasks and even when you sleep (some angina may occur when you sleep).

The Holter monitor records a continuous trace of your heart beats throughout the whole time you are wearing it, and is programmed to 'pick up' every abnormality during that time, from episodes of ischaemia to bursts of abnormal rhythm, to the odd missed beat. It can compare the episodes of ischaemia with your count of episodes of pain. The difference gives the numbers of attacks of 'silent' ischaemia, and gives an idea of the whole burden of ischaemia your heart is carrying, day and night.

Treadmill testing and Holter monitoring can detect people who are at relatively high risk of a serious heart attack. Cardiologists now recommend that everyone with angina under the age of 65 years, regardless of whether their symptoms are mild or severe (remember they often bear no relationship to the severity of your atheroma), should be offered these tests. For those aged over 65, the decision to put them to such discomfort depends on their general fitness and on how much their angina is interfering with their quality of life.

Echocardiography, thallium-201 scan and PET

Three other tests, echocardiography, thallium-201 scans and positron emission tomography (PET), should also be mentioned. They are an addition to treadmill testing, and are used to examine the heart as it beats, almost like a cine-film.

Echocardiography uses sound waves to show the structures of the heart, including the integrity of the heart valves and the way the heart walls move. Thallium-201 scans use the properties of a radioactive isotope to show up lack of blood supply to areas of heart muscle. They can measure the thickness of the heart walls, showing where they are thickened by hypertension, and where they have been thinned by the after-effects of a previous heart attack. Other radio-isotopes are being developed to replace thallium, and will be in use more generally in the near future.

PET, a complex combination of nuclear medicine techniques with multiple X-rays, can measure the blood flow through different areas of the heart. It can identify the effect that a particular stenosis has on the heart muscle beyond it, differentiating between muscle that is still working and areas of 'infarction' (muscle death). Of all these techniques, PET is the most accurate, but it is also the most expensive. It may not be in general use for the investigation of all angina cases for a long time.

Coronary angiography

Angiograms are just pictures of the inside of arteries. A small tube, or catheter, is fed from an artery in a leg or arm back up into the heart. Dye that shows up on X-ray is released into the openings of the coronary arteries, and as it fills the coronary system the progress is watched by the cardiologist as it happens. The circulation of the heart can be seen in minute detail.

Coronary angiography can pinpoint the sites of narrowing of the coronary arteries, and can suggest areas suitable for bypass surgery. When the results are assessed together with echocardiography, a thallium-201 (or other radio-isotope) scan, and PET, a complete picture of the problems of the heart is given. On the basis of that picture, the next step – treatment – will be decided.

These tests sound frightening, but they are not as bad as they seem, and the coronary unit staff will do their best to put you at your ease at every stage. These tests are important, and a full assessment of your particular problem cannot be made without them; so if you are offered them, please accept. They will help your doctors to make the best possible judgement on what is best for you.

12

Treating angina – medicines and surgery

The decision to treat your angina with drugs alone, or surgery to open up the coronary circulation, or both, depends on the results of the tests described in the last chapter.

Types of angina

The first decision that has to be made is on the urgency of your case. Angina is divided into three main forms – (1) stable, (2) unstable, and (3) variant (also called vasospastic or Prinzmetal).

In stable angina (1), there is usually a fixed stenosis of a particular segment of coronary artery that regularly leads to angina after the same amount of exercise is taken. If you have it, you get to know just how much you can do before the pain starts. It can be precipitated by exercise, emotional excitement (remember John Hunter in Chapter 1), or even by exposure to cold. Plunging the hands into cold water used to be a test for angina in the days before today's more scientific tests. Stable angina is predictable, and tends to be well managed by the patient. It is not an indication for priority treatment, unless the angiogram and scans show a very high immediate risk of complete blockage of the artery, or that the heart wall is very abnormal.

Unstable angina (2) is an emergency. It occurs unpredictably, sometimes even at rest, as well as during exercise. It can deteriorate very quickly, starting after less and less exercise over a few hours. It indicates that there is intermittent complete blockage of an artery, that may soon become permanent – leading to a myocardial infarction (heart attack).

The probable cause of unstable angina is a thrombus (a clot) in the artery, which may be based on excessive platelet activity. People with this form of angina must be admitted to a coronary care unit and treated immediately with anti-clotting (anticoagulant) drugs. They may even need emergency balloon angioplasty – a technique that is described later in this chapter.

Variant, vasospastic or Prinzmetal angina (3) can also be unpredictable, occurring without warning when the patient is resting. Paradoxically, it may disappear on exercise. Angiograms in Prinzmetal angina (it was named after the doctor who first described it) show no obstruction or stenoses, and very little evidence of atheroma. But when angiograms are done during an attack, they show that the coronary artery concerned is in spasm – a form of 'cramp' of the vessel wall muscles that leads to transient narrowing. Exercise relieves the spasm, and therefore the angina. Prinzmetal angina responds very well to the calcium antagonist group of drugs to be described later. If you have it, you will not need surgery.

One unusual form of angina diagnosed at this stage is 'syndrome X'. It is thus called because its cause is unknown, and it is also associated with 'clean' coronary arteries. However, the ECG does show that the angina pain is real, with ischaemic changes in areas of the heart on exercise. Patients with syndrome X have other problems: they have hypertension and a higher than normal blood glucose level, though not enough for them to be diagnosed as having diabetes. If you are found to have syndrome X, the aim of your treatment will be to bring your blood pressure and your blood glucose levels into their normal ranges. You will be advised on changes in your lifestyle and offered drug treatment for your hypertension, as well as the usual anti-angina treatment.

Treatment – drugs and surgery

The aim of all treatment of angina is to restore the balance of the supply–demand equation. Effective drugs must either improve the supply of oxygen to the myocardium, or reduce the heart's demand for it by decreasing its workload. Effective surgery aims to open up the coronary artery concerned either by stretching its walls and keeping them opened, or by creating a 'bypass' around the narrowed segment to maintain the flow of blood beyond it.

Drugs for angina

The three main classes of drug used are nitrates, beta-blockers and calcium antagonists:

Nitrates Nitrates relieve all forms of angina – stable, unstable and variant. For many years they have been known to work in angina, but it is only in the last three years or so that we know how they do it. The main substance that causes small blood vessels such as the coronary arteries to widen (dilate) is nitric oxide (NO). It is produced naturally by the lining cells of the arteries in response to changes in blood flow and in blood chemistry. Nitrates are converted in the blood to NO, and open up the blood vessels accordingly.

Their main effect is on the large veins, so that blood pools in the veins, and less returns to the heart. This lowers the pressure created inside the heart as it fills, which in turn lowers the tension in the walls of the heart, and therefore lowers the heart's oxygen needs. By opening up the smallest arteries in the periphery of the body – mainly in the limbs – nitrates also lower the force that the heart needs to exert on the circulation, and this too lowers the heart's oxygen needs. They also appear to distribute the coronary circulation to the areas of the heart, deep in the myocardium, that have been short of blood during angina attacks. In all three ways, they tend to return to normal the supply–demand equation.

Nitrates can be fast-acting or long-acting. Fast-acting ones such as *glyceryl trinitrate* are mainly used to stop angina attacks once they have begun. Glyceryl trinitrate is placed on or under the tongue or in the cheek as a spray, or as a tablet to be spat out as soon as the pain is relieved. Its effects are fastest when used under the tongue, and the pain relief is almost immediate. Some people use an under-the-tongue tablet just before exercise that they know will cause angina. This is only advisable in stable angina, when you know very well what to expect.

Longer-acting nitrates are used to prevent angina attacks. They include 'sustained release' forms of glyceryl trinitrate, and tablets (to be swallowed) of *pentaerythritol tetranitrate, isosorbide dinitrate* and *isosorbide mononitrate.*

Glyceryl trinitrate is well absorbed through the skin, and can be applied as an ointment or through a 'transdermal' patch that is stuck to the skin, like a sticking plaster. Many people stick the patch on their chest, but it would reach the heart just as fast if it were placed anywhere on the torso.

Side effects of nitrates include headache and facial flushing. Both are more common when you start the treatment, and usually fade with time. Unfortunately, the effects on angina sometimes fade too, so that the dose has to be increased. Do not increase the dose yourself without first discussing it with your doctor.

Beta-blockers Beta-blockers reduce the frequency and the severity of exercise-induced angina. They are *not* advised for Prinzmetal angina, which they can make even worse. They work by slowing and reducing the force of the heart beat, thereby diminishing the need of the heart for oxygen.

The slowing of the pulse can be dramatic, falling in some people to 50 beats per minute or below. If you feel well on that heart rate, do not worry – it will not do you any harm. However, beta-blockers do have side effects that you should know about if you are taking them. The most serious is a worsening of heart failure in people who have already had a heart attack, so patients should be carefully selected, by the tests mentioned in Chapter 11, before they are given them.

Also, a potentially serious side effect of beta-blockers is wheezing. People with a history of asthma can be pitched into a full-blown attack by a beta-blocker, so they are generally given another type of drug, such as a calcium antagonist (see below). However, beta-blockers may also stimulate wheezing in people who have never had asthma. So if you feel short of breath or wheezy after being prescribed a beta-blocker, report it to your doctor: it may not be the right drug for you.

Beta-blockers are divided into two main types – cardioselective drugs with less effect on the lung, and non-selective drugs that are more likely to cause wheezing. Among the first category are *acebutolol, atenolol, bisoprolol* and *metoprolol*. The second group contains *nadolol, oxprenolol, pindolol, propranolol, sotalol* and *timolol*. If you find a drug from the second group has made you wheezy, you can try one from the first, but you still need to take care if you have had asthma in the past.

Other beta-blocker side effects include lethargy, bad dreams, a fuzzy head, inability to concentrate and cold feet. One serious side effect that I suspect affects more men than the reports suggest is impotence. If you find that you are impotent on a beta-blocker, don't blame it on your heart, and don't suffer in silence. You may return to normal with a change of drug.

Calcium antagonists Calcium antagonists, also known as calcium entry blockers, act by blocking the inward movement of calcium into cells. This causes the small blood vessels in the limbs to dilate, lowering blood pressure; it dilates the coronary arteries, increasing the oxygen supply to the heart muscle; and it makes the heart muscle itself more efficient, so that its demand for oxygen at any level of exercise is reduced. Calcium antagonists therefore improve the supply–demand equation in several ways. They allow you to exercise longer and harder before the onset of angina as a result of exertion, and they prevent the spasm of Prinzmetal angina.

However, not all calcium antagonists act in the same way. They have been classified into three groups. The first group includes *verapamil*, which depresses the function of the heart, making the beat weaker and slower. This is important, as it can cause heart failure if it is given along with a beta-blocker, or if there is a particular type of abnormal heart rhythm.

In the second group are *amlodipine, nicardipine* and *nifedipine*. They do not depress the heart: in fact, they may reverse some of the cardiac-slowing effects of beta-blockers, and can be prescribed with them, as long as the blood pressure is watched very closely – given together, they can lower blood pressure too far.

The third group of calcium antagonists includes *diltiazem*, which has no cardiac-stimulating or depressing effect, and is neither dangerous nor helpful with a beta-blocker.

Nitrates and calcium antagonists of the second group may be prescribed together in some patients with both angina and a degree of heart failure, or with certain heart rhythm disturbances.

Side effects of calcium antagonists include palpitations and flushing, but for the most part they are relatively free of side effects. One problem for them has been that in their original tablet or capsule forms they were relatively short acting, so that the effect lasted only a few hours. This could be bad for patients, because there were periods of many hours in each day in which they were not protected by their drug.

This has changed with *amlodipine*, which has a longer action, and covers most of the day and night. Nifedipine too has been introduced in a once-daily form that acts for 24 hours. This is a very important step forward, particularly when the angina is linked with hypertension, as the once-daily dose of *Nifedipine LA*, or *Nifedipine GITS*, deals effectively with that too.

If you are given a prescription for a long-acting calcium antagonist like Nifedipine LA, do not accept any other nifedipine preparation as a substitute, as it will not work in the same way. This is one area of medicine in which the brand name matters, and the 'generic' preparations are *not* the same.

Potassium channel activators These are a new class of drug, the first of which is *nicorandil*. Their main action is, like nitrates, to dilate small arteries and veins. However, their action, unlike nitrates, does not appear to fade with time. Nicorandil increases the flow of blood through the coronary arteries, even in areas beyond stenoses. It can be used alone or combined with other anti-angina drugs. It does not depress the heart or have any effect on blood pressure or heart rate in people with angina.

Aspirin No review of drugs used for angina would be complete without a mention of aspirin. In these circumstances, aspirin is not being prescribed for its well-known effect on pain, but for its effect on the platelets in the bloodstream. In low doses, half a standard aspirin tablet per day, aspirin prevents platelets from sticking together or from adhering to the surface of atheromatous plaques.

As this is the first step to thrombosis at the site of a plaque, aspirin should, in theory, prevent the thromboses within the coronary arteries at stenotic sites that are thought to be the main cause of heart attacks. The whole medical world now accepts, after many trials have shown its effects, that one aspirin should be given at the time of an acute heart attack to minimize the damage, and thereafter to prevent a further attack.

It is a very small step from giving such a low dose of aspirin during a heart attack to its use to prevent one in people with angina. I advise all my patients with angina to take half an aspirin a day. The very few who cannot tolerate this dose of the drug because it gives them indigestion may have to do without it, but it is possibly a life-saver for the rest. It has no obvious effect on the angina, but it may well prevent the angina from becoming a full-blown heart attack.

Lowering cholesterol The general feeling among doctors is that people with angina should take their own action – such as eating healthily, stopping smoking and exercising regularly – to lower their blood cholesterol levels, and that very few actually need drugs to do the job for them.

This is not because the drugs do not work. They do, very successfully, lower blood lipid (fat) levels. However, there is very little proof that they actually benefit patients, because the trials of lipid-lowering drugs have had equivocal results. Because of this, the British Hyperlipidaemia Association (BHA) (which is concerned with diseases in which the blood levels of fats are raised) and the European Atherosclerosis Society (EAS) have laid down guidelines to doctors about prescribing such drugs for people with higher than normal levels of cholesterol and other related lipids in the blood.

The BHA and EAS stress very strongly that cholesterol-lowering drugs should not be considered until other risk factors for atheroma have been controlled or eliminated. They list the most important of them as being smoking, alcohol consumption, obesity, diabetes, hypertension and physical inactivity.

They then advise that people with total cholesterol levels above 5.2 mmol/l but below 6.5 mmol/l should receive dietary counselling involving the general principles of weight reduction, a diet low in saturated fat and cholesterol, and high in fibre.

Those with cholesterol levels above 6.5 mmol/l but below 7.8 mmol/l should be given a thorough trial of diet, which will be effective for most of them. If they do not respond with a good reduction in cholesterol, especially if they have other risk factors such as hypertension and a previous heart attack, then drug treatment should be considered.

For those with cholesterol levels above 7.8 mmol/l, diet is still essential, but the majority will need drugs. Most people with this level of blood cholesterol have inherited their condition (familial hypercholesterolaemia): they may need two drugs with different actions to lower their levels satisfactorily.

Lipid-lowering drugs

A high blood level of fat – the correct medical term for it is 'hyperlipidaemia' – is a broad term covering several conditions in which one or other of the different types of fat in the blood is raised. I have referred throughout the book to cholesterol, but this is a simplification. In fact, there are at least five different forms of hyperlipidaemia, and different types of lipid-lowering drugs are needed to correct them. Among them are:

- Bile acid sequestrants
- Nicotinic acid derivatives
- Fibrates
- Statins

Bile acid sequestrants Bile acid sequestrants such as *cholestyramine* and *colestipol* act by increasing the breakdown of cholesterol in the liver, which in turn leads to lower blood cholesterol levels. However, they only reduce 'LDL cholesterol' – one fraction of the total blood cholesterol.

Here it may be helpful to explain the jargon around cholesterol and blood lipids. Cholesterol and triglycerides, the two prominent fats, or lipids, are carried around in the bloodstream by 'lipoproteins' – combinations of protein and fat. The lipoproteins are classified according to their densities, so that low-density lipoproteins are LDL, intermediate-density lipoproteins are IDL, high-density lipoproteins are HDL, and very low-density lipoproteins are VLDL.

The higher the LDL in the blood, the greater the risk of angina and heart attack – it seems that LDL is the substance that carries the cholesterol and triglycerides into the atheromatous plaques. In contrast, the higher the HDL, the lower the risk of heart attack. HDL seems to 'carry away' the cholesterol from the bloodstream into the liver, where it is broken down into bile acids and excreted in the faeces. VLDL does not appear to affect coronary risk much, if at all: IDL may make it worse, but LDL is the main villain.

Because they only reduce LDL, the bile acid sequestrants are only prescribed for patients known to have a high LDL cholesterol level – known as 'Type 2' hyperlipidaemia. They are not used in hyperlipidaemias due to rises in other forms of lipids such as triglycerides. As cholestyramine and colestipol decrease the absorption of vitamins A, D and K from food, they must be given as a food supplement if you are taking them for a long time. They may also interfere with the absorption of other drugs, so they should be taken at least an hour before them.

Probucol, although not strictly a bile acid sequestrant, has similar results to cholestyramine and colestipol, in that it increases the excretion of cholesterol in the bile. It, too, should only be used in Type 2 hyperlipidaemia. It persists for many weeks in fatty tissues, and should be stopped at least six months before a planned pregnancy.

Nicotinic acid derivatives These not only lower LDL levels, but they also lower blood levels of other lipid fractions, such as VLDL and IDL, and triglycerides. They can therefore be used in Types 2, 4 and 5 hyperlipidaemias, in which the triglyceride levels are raised, along with LDL, VLDL and IDL cholesterol. *Nicotinic acid* itself causes intense flushing and headache, but this can be reduced by starting with a lower dose. Some experts prefer to ask their patients to tolerate the side effects from the start, on the basis that they always subside even when you continue with the drug, and the higher starting dose is beneficial from the beginning of treatment.

Acipimox is a nicotinic acid derivative that is claimed not only to decrease LDL and VLDL, but also to increase HDL. This would be a considerable benefit.

Fibrates Fibrates reduce plasma triglycerides and VLDL, and increase HDL. However, they can cause muscle pains as a result of toxic effects on the muscles themselves, especially if they are given along with statins (see below). People taking fibrates must have a regular blood test for a substance called creatine phosphokinase (CPK), a rise in which pre-dates the muscle pains. They should be asked to report any episode of muscle pain.

The fibrates include *bezafibrate, clofibrate, ciprofibrate, fenofibrate* and *gemfibrozil*. The choice of which fibrate to prescribe depends on the type of hyperlipidaemia you have, and you should be guided by your specialist on which to take, or whether you take them at all. A risk with clofibrate, but apparently not with the other fibrates, is that it may concentrate the bile so much that it causes gallstones.

Statins These include *fluvastatin, pravastatin* and *simvastatin*. They are all prescribed for people with a blood cholesterol of 6.5 mmol/l or above. They block the liver's ability to make cholesterol, reducing

LDL levels by as much as 40 per cent, decreasing triglyceride levels to a lesser degree, and raising the beneficial HDL levels. Like fibrates, all statins can cause muscle pains and weakness, and CPK levels must be measured regularly when people are taking them.

Marine triglycerides Marine triglycerides such as *Maxepa* reduce LDL cholesterol and triglycerides, probably by reducing their production in the liver. They have the extra bonus of shifting the balance of platelet activity away from aggregation and thrombosis, so that they reduce the risk of a thrombosis inside a coronary artery.

This action is probably why eating three oily fish meals a week appears to reduce the risk of a heart attack. Oily fish means mackerel, herring, sardines, pilchards, trout and salmon. Their fats and triglycerides differ structurally from the fat of land animals, with the fish oils appearing to protect against atheroma and thrombosis. The Inuit people, whose meat is almost entirely derived from marine animals and fish, have a very low heart attack rate.

When surgery is needed in angina – bypass, angioplasty, lasers and stents

In the early 1980s, cardiologists were still arguing as to whether bypass surgery to improve the coronary artery flow was worthwhile. There were doubts about its safety and its long-term benefits. In the early days, many bypasses closed off a few months after the operation, leaving the patients no better off.

These doubts are now dispelled. Bypass surgery is now accepted as improving the quality of life of thousands of angina sufferers, and as saving many lives. It has a very high success rate, and the 're-stenosis' rate (when the new artery closes off) is diminishing year by year.

To bypass surgery has been added balloon angioplasty and, more recently, laser and stent treatment.

Bypass surgery When bypass surgery was first started, it was usual to take a vein from the leg (we have plenty to spare!) and insert it around the narrowed site in the coronary artery. The blood then flows through the vein, around the stenosis, to reach the myocardium beyond it. The immediate result is a much better flow of blood to the heart muscle, carrying much more oxygen and glucose to the 'starved' area.

There has been a more recent trend to use a small segment of artery from inside the chest wall – the internal mammary artery – instead of the vein. Among the reasons for the change is that the artery is more readily available than a leg vein, and that an arterial graft is probably more appropriate than a vein graft for what after all is another artery. There have been reports that the internal mammary graft is more effective in the long term, but other comparisons between the two seem to suggest that there is little difference in the merits of the two types of graft.

Bypass grafts are, of course, done under general anaesthetic, and patients must stay in hospital for several days afterwards. I was astonished to be called to a patient's home on a Friday to see him, to be told that he had had his bypass just four days before, on the Monday! The pressure to remove patients from hospital care in Britain's 'marketplace' health service is surely immense!

Bypass surgery is mostly used when there are multiple small blockages of one, two or all three coronary arteries, and where the blockages are in vessels too small for angioplasty to be attempted.

Balloon angioplasty Angioplasty means changing the shape of a blood vessel. In balloon angioplasty a thin catheter is passed through an artery in the leg up the main artery in the abdomen, the aorta, into the heart, and the tip inserted into the affected coronary artery, under X-ray control.

The tip of the catheter is passed through the narrowed section (which has been identified by a previous coronary angiogram). Just short of the tip the catheter forms a tiny balloon, which is inflated once it is exactly opposite the narrowed segment of artery. This compresses the atheromatous plaque back into the wall of the artery, widening it. After angioplasty, the blood flow through that section of artery is usually multiplied many times.

Original doubts about angioplasty have been cast aside, now that many thousands of people have been treated, and the successes have been obvious. It has a greater than 90 per cent success rate in coronary arteries, and many angina patients feel much better immediately after it is done.

Angioplasty is performed under local anaesthesia and moderate sedation, so that you will be hazily conscious throughout it. It is performed in the operating theatre, however, with an anaesthetist on hand, so that on the very rare occasions that the catheter causes angina, the team can swing into a full bypass operation.

Stents and lasers To balloons and bypasses have now been added stents and lasers. The catheter technology that uses balloons can also put stents in place. Stents are tiny tubes, made up of what looks like wire mesh, that can be placed in the narrowed section of artery to keep it open. The stent is placed there in a folded or collapsed form, and springs open when it is released at the right spot. It can be left there permanently, as the lining of the blood vessel grows around the mesh, holding it in place, and at the same time remaining wide open.

The catheter technology is also being developed to use lasers to 'burn away' plaques that protrude into the bloodstream, under direct vision. This is still a research procedure, but it cannot be long before it becomes one of the choices for the cardiologist.

The results Thousands of people have now enjoyed more than ten years of very full active lives after bypass and angioplasty operations. Their lives have been changed beyond belief. The benefits, however, cannot be put down entirely to their surgery. The ones who have done best are those who changed many other aspects of their lives too.

They stopped smoking, controlled their drinking, changed their eating habits, exercised more, lost their excess weight, and adopted an altogether new lifestyle. Their hospital treatment offered them a chance to start life again, and they took it. This must be the definitive and lasting message for everyone with angina.

13
Women – and children

In the summer television season in Britain in 1995, a series of weekly programmes about women's health was shown. Called *The Lady-killers*, it concentrated on the diseases that the producers felt were killing women in the last decade of the twentieth century. It highlighted cervical, ovarian and breast cancer, post-natal depression, rheumatoid arthritis, ectopic pregnancy and pregnancy toxaemia. These are all very worthwhile disorders to show, but they fade into insignificance when compared with the deaths in women as a result of heart disease.

Women and angina and heart disease

Coronary artery disease is now the most common cause of death in women in most developed countries, including Britain and the United States. This is mainly because the coronary death rate rises steeply after the menopause: by the age of 65, as many women as men are dying from heart attacks; and over the age of 80, heart attacks are much commoner in women, proportionately, than in men.

However, heart attacks do occur in much younger women: of the deaths caused by heart attacks in women aged under 65, one in four is in a woman aged under 45. Therefore it is clear that women and their doctors must know their risks and try to avoid them.

The research results

There is plenty of evidence that many heart problems in women go unsuspected by themselves and undiagnosed by their doctors – and three papers in the *British Medical Journal* on 3 September 1994 make that clear. Dr Karen Clarke and her team at Nottingham University found that women in their area with severe chest pain took longer to arrive in hospital, were less likely than men to be admitted to acute coronary care, were less likely to receive the life-saving antithrombotic treatments, had more severe heart damage, were more ill, and were slightly more likely to die in hospital! Furthermore, after their heart attacks they were less likely to be given aspirin and beta-blocker treatment when they went home. Dr Clarke and her researchers concluded that women were not getting a fair deal.

Dr Paul Wilkinson's group at the London School of Hygiene and Tropical Medicine came to the same conclusion after following the treatment of people admitted to coronary care in London from 1988 to 1992. After six months, 63 per cent of the women, and 76 per cent of the men, were still alive – and this difference could not be attributed to an age difference. Dr Wilkinson concluded that the women had less vigorous treatment for their heart problems than did the men. He asked for effective strategies to be developed to protect women during the early period after a heart attack.

In the third *British Medical Journal* paper, Philip Hannaford, Clifford Kay and Susan Ferry, of the Manchester Research Unit of the Royal College of General Practitioners, wrote that many cardiologists operated a policy of not giving older patients anti-clotting therapy in the acute phase of heart attacks – and that women were more likely than men to fall into that category. Hence the higher failure rate with women.

The difference between the sexes does not end with the treatment of heart attacks, though – it applies to angina too. M.A. Pfeffer, an American physician, found that twice as many men as women with angina were given angiography and bypass grafts, even though the severity of their angina was the same. J.N. Tobin found that men with angina who had abnormal heart movement scans were ten times more likely to be given angiography than women with similar problems. They were also four times more likely to be given coronary bypass surgery than women with the same coronary artery abnormality.

So it is very clear that women with angina are losing out all round. They are being offered less effective treatment of their angina; and when they actually have heart attacks, they are more likely to die than men because they are not given the same potentially life-saving treatment.

This makes me very angry, and I am not a woman – so if you are female, you have every right to be furious! What you can do about it is spelled out below.

Steps that women can take to protect their hearts

First, it is true that women who develop heart attacks tend to be older than their male counterparts; and they are at more risk from heart attacks if they have high blood pressure and diabetes. So if you have one or other, or both, of these conditions (they often go together), you *must* be particularly careful to keep them under good control.

For high blood pressure, that means taking the correct anti-hypertensive drugs and having monthly blood pressure checks. For diabetes, it means strict control of weight – the BMI (Body Mass Index) should be strictly between 20 and 25, and preferably closer to the lower figure. Small meals containing large amounts of fibre, taken frequently, with multiple injections of small amounts of insulin each day, a daily diary card of your blood glucose, and a monthly visit to your diabetic clinic are all essentials.

The female hormone oestrogen appears to protect women against heart attacks – a protection that falls away after the menopause. So why not try hormone replacement therapy (HRT) after your menopause, to keep your heart attack risk low? In a large study of American nurses, HRT halved the risk of coronary disease in post-menopausal women. Worries that HRT might cause breast cancer appear to be unfounded, but there is very definite evidence that it greatly reduces the risk of ovarian cancer – and also, surprisingly, of rheumatoid arthritis. Nevertheless, women with many close relatives with breast cancer should probably avoid HRT: there may be a very small risk that it can accelerate the development of an already existing growth.

The good news for women about heart disease is that the very strong risk in men with high cholesterol levels probably does not apply to women. Younger women naturally have higher blood cholesterol levels than men of the same age, but most of it is of the beneficial HDL type. Only if there is obvious hyperlipidaemia, or a history of early deaths from heart attacks in women in the immediate family, should a high cholesterol level in a woman be taken as worrying, and needing a special diet or drugs.

The dangers for women who continue to smoke

The bad news is that women are continuing to smoke, and younger women are taking it up more readily than did their mothers at the same age. Forty per cent of teenage girls, but only 30 per cent of teenage boys, are reported to be smokers.

For women who smoke, the facts are simple:

- Pre-menopausal smokers have three times the heart attack rate of their non-smoker colleagues.
- Women smoking more than 40 cigarettes a day increase their heart attack risk by 20-fold.
- Combining smoking with diabetes hugely increases the heart attack risk in women, well above that in similar men.
- Oral contraceptive users who smoke heavily increase their risk of thrombosis in the pelvis, legs and brain. The risk rises very steeply from their mid-thirties onwards.

Surgery for women with angina

Women with angina who are offered a coronary artery bypass operation should accept the chance. Even though they tend naturally to have narrower coronary arteries than men, the results of bypass grafts in women and men are equally good. Women with angina who have never had a heart attack do even better after bypass surgery than similar men.

So go for it, ladies! Your doctors have been alerted to the fact that you have had a raw deal, and need to be treated more vigorously.

For your own part, recognize that you are at risk by not ignoring that pain in your chest. Do not smoke – *at all*. Have regular health checks. If you have high blood pressure and/or diabetes, be meticulous about their control. And try to keep to a normal weight – not overweight, but not too thin either. Most models in women's magazines are far too thin, and anorexia kills faster than atheroma! Finally, if you are menopausal or older, do consider HRT. It could do your heart a lot of good.

Children and angina

Why should children feature in this book? They are at the other end of life, after all, from the years of angina. Yet, shockingly, they are already on their way towards it. Many experts in heart disease are fearful for the future of this generation of schoolchildren.

Think of the changes in society that are pushing children towards heart disease. They no longer walk to school, because of parents' fears of letting youngsters walk alone in our dangerous streets. At school they no longer have school lunches, but often eat junk food in cafés instead. Teachers no longer wish to organize games and sports for them, so they never get into the habit of regular exercise for fun. Physical education lessons amount to less than two 30-minute periods a week – and often these seem less vigorous than a generation ago. At the last school PE period I witnessed, half the children had clipboards monitoring the other half's exercise! In the Thatcher years in Britain, thousands of acres of school playing fields were sold off to provide short-term profits for the Treasury. What a short-sighted policy!

One of these changes would be worrying in itself, but all of them together make a nightmare that will arrive in the early years of the next century. Heart disease rates have been falling in many countries as people have accepted the health message. Does the next generation have to learn again, the hard way? If you have children in your home, whose lifestyles you recognize from the last few paragraphs, please take some time to discuss these things with them. Most *do* listen, even if they may not at first.

I cannot finish this book, however, on a 'down' note. I keep remembering the day of the Great Scottish Run, in August 1995. Some 3,000 children turned out to run for 3 kilometres through Glasgow Green – a park in the centre of Scotland's biggest city. Around 10,000 parents and friends turned out to watch them.

Then 7,200 adults ran the half-marathon through the city streets. All but a few professional runners were taking part to benefit medical and health-based charities. It seemed the whole of Glasgow came to watch us as we struggled in the 90 degree heat. With that sort of enthusiasm for the best efforts of our fellow man, surely the next generation will get things right.

Appendix 1:
Useful Organizations

Action on Smoking and Health (ASH)
109 Gloucester Place,
London
W1H 3PH
Tel: 0171–935 3519

British Heart Foundation
14 Fitzhardinge Street
London
W1H 4DH
Tel: 0171–953 0185

Chest, Heart and Stroke, Scotland
65 North Castle Street
Edinburgh
EH2 3LT
Tel: 0131–225 6963

Appendix 2:

Glossary

ACE inhibitor A type of drug sometimes used to reduce high blood pressure.

Angina pectoris Pain in the chest, usually due to failure of the flow of blood to the heart to meet the heart's demands for oxygen and glucose.

Angiogram An X-ray procedure to show the circulation through an artery.

Angioplasty An operation, usually using a balloon on a catheter, to flatten an atherosclerotic plaque that is intruding into the inside – into the blood stream – of a coronary artery.

Artery A blood vessel leading from the heart to the rest of the body. (A vein leads to the heart from the rest of the body.)

Atheroma, atherosclerosis A degenerative condition of the arteries that can lead to angina.

Autonomic nervous system The system of nerves that controls the function of the muscles used in digestion, the circulation, breathing, etc.

Beta-blocker A drug that blocks a specific part of the action of the autonomic nervous system. It slows the heart and reduces the force of the heart beat.

Blood pressure The pressure at which the blood circulates in the arteries. It has two components – systolic and diastolic pressures.

Bypass surgery An operation that fits another healthy blood vessel around the site of a narrowed coronary artery.

Calcium antagonist A type of drug to lower blood pressure and to ease angina.

Carbon monoxide Poisonous gas that displaces oxygen from red blood cells, thereby greatly increasing the risk of angina and heart attack. Greatly raised in smokers' blood.

Cholesterol Fatty material that circulates in the blood. In atheroma it is abnormally deposited on the inside surfaces of arteries. (See fatty streaks.)

Coronary artery One of three arteries that take blood from inside the heart (that has been fully oxygenated in the lungs) to 'feed' the myocardium (the heart muscle) with oxygen and glucose.

Coronary thrombosis A clot of blood in a coronary artery. This can lead to myocardial infarction (see under).

Echocardiogram A method of examining the heart using ultrasound waves. It can show how the heart wall and valves move with each beat.

Electrocardiogram (ECG) A device to display the electrical activity of the heart on a chart. It can show whether there is a cardiac cause for angina pectoris.

Fatty streaks The earliest signs of atherosclerosis.

Fibrinogen A substance in the bloodstream that promotes thrombosis (see under). Greatly increased in smokers.

Glucose The sugar upon which all energy processes in every cell in the body depends.

HDL High density lipoprotein. This substance carries away cholesterol from the arteries into the liver to be excreted – so that the higher the HDL in the bloodstream, the better.

Holter testing Use of a portable ECG machine to monitor the function of the heart for up to 48 hours.

Hypertension High blood pressure. It can consist of raised systolic pressure, raised diastolic pressure, or both.

Infarction Death of any tissue due to lack of blood supply to it.

Ischaemia A relative lack of blood supply. The heart becomes ischaemic if not enough blood is flowing through the coronary arteries to sustain the work being done.

Lipoproteins Substances that carry fats such as cholesterol around the body in the bloodstream.

LDL Low density lipoprotein. This carries cholesterol from the bloodstream into the blood vessel wall, so that the higher its level, the greater the risk of atherosclerosis.

Myocardial infarction Death of a part of the myocardium due to complete blockage of the blood flow to it. Commonly known as a heart attack.

Myocardium The heart muscle.

Nicotine Poison that narrows arteries and causes abnormal heartbeats. Inhaled in cigarette smoke.

Nitrate Drug that opens up blood vessels, thereby improving the blood flow through them.

Plaque A plate-like thickened area on the inside surface of an artery, caused by atherosclerosis.

Platelets Tiny fragments of cells in the bloodstream which, when they stick together ('aggregate'), can initiate a thrombosis in an artery. Aspirin in low dose (a quarter tablet a day) is a platelet 'anti-aggregating agent', thereby preventing thrombosis.

Radio-isotope scan A system of detecting areas of heart muscle that are not working properly. Often uses Caesium.

Stenosis A site of narrowing of a coronary artery, so that the blood flow through it is much diminished.

Thrombosis Clotting of blood within a blood vessel. In a coronary artery, it is coronary thrombosis, which is the cause of most heart attacks or myocardial infarctions.

Treadmill A moving 'pavement' used to measure the exercise a person needs to perform to provoke an angina attack.

Triglycerides A fatty material, high levels of which are linked with atherosclerosis.

Index

acipimox 102
Action on Smoking and Health (ASH) 78
aerobic exercise 61–2
alcohol 81–5
angioplasty 104
aspirin 99
atheroma 21–3

Beevers, Dr Gareth 82–3
betablockers 97
blood pressure 36, 86–8
Body Mass Index (BMI) 33–6, 54, 108
British Hyperlipidaemia Association 100
British Regional Heart Study 1, 32–3, 38–9
Buerger's disease 28
bypass surgery 103–4

calcium antagonists 97–9
carbon monoxide 23–5, 28
children 109–10
cholesterol 24, 33, 36–8, 40–9
cholestyramine 47, 101
Clarke, Dr Karen 106
clofibrate 45, 47
colestipol 101
coronary angiography 92

coronary arteries 20
cotinine 51

Darwin, Charles 56
diabetes 87–8
drugs for angina 99–103

eating well 51–4
echocardiography 92
electrocardiogram (ECG) 7, 9, 10, 89–92
European Atherosclerosis Society 100
Exercise 55–69

fibrates 102
fibrinogen 26–7
Finnish Mental Hospitals Study 43
Fixx, Jim 8–9, 55
Framingham Study 32

Gaulle, General de 76
Great Scottish Run 7, 58, 110

Harvard Step Test 58-60, 69
Haviland, Dr 33, 69
HDL 101, 108
holter monitoring 91
hormone replacement therapy

(HRT) 108
Hunter, John 7–8

IDL 101
infarction 20
International Atherosclerosis
    Project 31
ischaemic heart disease 15
Isles, Dr Christopher 42

Jane 9–10
Japanese 22
Jim 5–7

Kaiser Permanente Study 84
Kavanagh, Dr Terence 68
Keys, Professor Ancel 31
King's College Hospital 81, 84

lactic acid 20
lasers 105
LDL 101
linoleic acid 37
lipid-lowering drugs 100–3
Lipids Research Clinics Study
    46–7
lipoproteins 24
*Living with High Blood
    Pressure* (1995) 88
Los Angeles Veterans
    Administration Study 43

Manchester Research Unit 107
Mancia, Professor Giuseppe
    86–7
Mann, Dr G. V. 48–9
marathons and half marathons
    68–9

marine triglycerides 103
Mediterranean diet 37, 52–5
MONICA 41
MRFIT 45
myocardium 18

nicotine 70–80
nicotinic acid 102
Nifedipine LA 99
Nightingale, Florence 56
nitrates 89, 95–6
North Karelia Project 32, 43
Norway 29–30, 40

oesophagus, spasm of 13
Oliver, Professor Michael 37,
    52
Oslo Study Group 46
osteoporosis 68

pernicious anaemia 12
Pfeffer, Dr M. A. 107
position emission tomography
    (PET) 92
potassium channel activators 99
prinzmetal angina 94
probucol 102

red blood cells 25
relaxation 66–7
rosemary 12
running 62

Seven Countries Study 31–2
Shaper, Professor A. G. 39, 83
SHEP Study 87
smoking 27–8, 34, 51, 70–80
statins 102

stents 105
Sunday Mail 58, 78
Surgery for angina 103–5; for
    women 109
syndrome X 95

Tai Chi 67
Thallium-201 scans 92
thrombosis 23
Tobin, Dr J. N. 107
treadmill testing 6, 91
Tunstall-Pedoe, Professor Hugh
    30, 42

United States – obesity trends 3

United Kingdom Medical
    Research Council Trial 88
unstable angina 94

variant angina 94
Veritas Society 48–9
VLDL 101

WHO European Collaborative
    Trial 44–5
Wilkinson, Dr Paul 107
Williams, Professor Roger 81
Wissler, Professor R. W. 40
women 58, 106–9

yoga 67